Intermittent Fasting: 2 Books in 1

This book includes: Autophagy and Intermittent fasting for Women. A Guide to Weight Loss, Burn Fat, Live Healthier Through the Metabolic Process of Autophagy

Written By

Rachel Dash

By reading this document, the reader agrees that under no circumstances is the author responsible for any losses, direct or indirect, which are incurred as a result of the use of information contained within this document, including, but not limited to, — errors, omissions, or inaccuracies.

Autophagy

Discover How to Live Healthy and Longer with Your Self-Cleansing Body's Natural Intelligence. Start a Fasting Diet Activating the Anti-Aging Process to Lose Weight Safely

(Pg 1)

Intermittent Fasting for Women

The A-Z Guide to Weight Loss, Burn Fat and Live Healthier Through the Process of Autophagy. Heal Your Body with an Intermittent, Alternate-Day and Extended Fasting Diet

(Pg 127)

Autophagy

Discover How to Live Healthy and Longer with Your Self-Cleansing Body's Natural Intelligence. Start a Fasting Diet Activating the Anti-Aging Process to Lose Weight Safely

Written By

Rachel Dash

By reading this document, the reader agrees that under no circumstances is the author responsible for any losses, direct or indirect, which are incurred as a result of the use of information contained within this document, including, but not limited to, — errors, omissions, or inaccuracies.

Table of Contents

Introduction

Thank you for purchasing *Autophagy: Discover How to Live Healthy and Longer with Your Self-Cleansing Body's Natural Intelligence.* In this book, you will learn about Autophagy and all of the health benefits that it has to offer. These benefits are numerous and include weight loss, increased energy, improved immune system functioning, and cancer-fighting ability. Yet the good things autophagy can do for you extend far beyond these and they will be explored specifically in order to help you better understand how you can improve your life by tapping into this important and natural cellular process. It is not as difficult as you might think.

Autophagy has become a buzz word in the health and fitness industry, much like the Atkins Diet and Keto. Like many other buzz words, autophagy is a term that many people are exposed to but relatively few understand. Autophagy is generally thought of as being similar to the more familiar apoptosis, which many will have learned about in school. But autophagy is quite from different this other major form of cell death, and it is this difference that will help you improve your health and wellbeing with this pathway. As you will discover, intermittent fasting, water fasting, fasting-mimicking, and other diets can stimulate autophagy and, as a result, lead to improved health outcomes and longevity.

Autophagy is how the body engages in the survival of the fittest on a cellular level. Autophagy allows the human body to consume and recycle components for a variety of purposes. These components can be used to build new cells or for energy. This process can be activated in many different ways, of which among the more common is through a protein called AMP-activated protein kinase, or AMPK. AMP Kinase is, in fact, an enzyme that plays an important role in energy conservation and homeostasis in the human body.

AMP Kinase is generated in situations when the body needs to metabolize its own components for

energy, as is the case when you are fasting both intentionally or simply because it is early in the day and you have not eaten yet. This is an important concept that will be explored in the book. Fasting can be something that you do deliberately over a long period, or it can be incorporated into periods in your day as part of a periodic fasting regime (i.e. intermittent fasting). As you will discover, many processes or foods can be used to stimulate autophagy for beneficial reasons.

For instance, much research has focused on foods that can play a role in stimulating autophagy for the purposes of fighting cancer or discouraging diseases. Many men and women choose to incorporate these types of foods into their diets even though they are not facing the ravages of cancer or another serious disease. The Reishi mushroom has been studied because of the role it plays in the suppression of colon cancer cell growth through the phosphorylation of a version of AMP Kinase. Green tea and ginger have also been studied because of their proven effects in cancer suppression by way of compounds EGCG and 6-Shagaal, respectively.

The human body does not really distinguish between fasting and starvation. Part of the reason why fasting works so well in stimulating autophagy is that the human body is always preparing for the worst. If you have not eaten for a prolonged period, your body realizes that it does not make sense to waste energy and other resources on components that are not contributing to the overall survival of the organism. This allows the body to use fasting, exercise and even reduced oxygen as triggers for autophagy. Stimulating autophagy, therefore, is nothing more than taking advantage of how your body has evolved to deal with stress and to survive.

Stimulation of autophagy, or Autophagy as it is conceptualized in this book, requires an understanding of what autophagy is and why it is. Autophagy is a type of cell death, and it is critical for it to be distinguished from the better-known apoptosis. Apoptosis is programmed cell death, which makes autophagy a form of non-programmed cell death. This has led to some perceiving autophagy as a haphazard process that represents sort of a "blue screen of death" for the body's cells, but nothing could be further from the truth.

Autophagy is how the body streamlines itself, a concept that will be further explored in the first two chapters. When we speak of survival of the fittest in the context of autophagy, what we mean is that sometimes the body finds it necessary to remove some components and encourage others. This happens on a molecular and cellular level through processes like autophagy. Autophagy allows the body to acutely and in a highly-controlled fashion remove cells that no longer align with the body's needs.

This sort of process can be essential to the survival of an organism, which is a major reason why autophagy has evolved to become a normal process in humans. Indeed, one of the goals of this book is to teach you how you can use this natural process of the body to lose weight, target fat, reduce your chances of cancer or other health ailments, and improve your wellbeing. Autophagy (as well as the specific processes that fall under its scope) is not a fad diet. This is a scientifically proven, normal process whose study has resulted in the awarding of a Nobel Prize (the most recent of which was in 2016).

Why is autophagy significant enough to award a scientist a Nobel Prize for its study? Research has found that doctors can use compounds isolated from plants to stimulate autophagy against cancer cells. Cancer is by definition the unregulated and dysfunctional growth of cells and tissues that eventually leads to death. Cancer cells cause damage to the organs where they form. Cancer cells eventually metastasize (or spread) to other tissues, leading to organ failure and eventual demise. Cell death is how the human body normally deals with dysfunctional cells. In particular, autophagy is the process that would allow the body to acutely remove cellular components through activation or up-regulation of proteins like AMP Kinase. The body's ultimate goal is to remove cells before they become cancerous, but no one is perfect and sometimes our bodies fail in this pursuit.

If scientists can tap into autophagy in states of cancer, then they may be able to reverse the cancer growth (or destroy the cells) without risking damaging normal tissues as happens with chemotherapy and radiation therapy. These types of treatments are regarded with fear by many because of the symptoms and side effects that stem from damage to normal cells during the attempt to eradicate the abnormal ones. But by tapping into natural autophagy processes, the human body would be able to breakdown these cancerous growths in an organized and systematic fashion without affecting the body's normal machinery.

This is part of what distinguishes autophagy from apoptosis, an important distinction that will be detailed at length in this book. This is a critical line to draw in your head because co-opting Autophagy will allow you to live a healthy and vigorous life, free from obesity and disease, while apoptosis would represent premature death of tissues. It may help to remember the word premature in the context of apoptosis as this will allow you to distinguish it from autophagy which is generally not premature, but ordered and necessary.

Because autophagy is thrown around so much on the internet, it is important to have a deep understanding of what it is on both the cellular and tissue level, which will be accomplished in the first and second chapters. Because of how autophagy works to recycle and remove redundant or problematic cellular components, the uses and advantages of autophagy tend to focus on certain areas. Autophagy can be used to reduce inflammation, stimulate anti-aging effects, improve immune function, improve brain function, provide protection from neurodegenerative diseases, and help men and women to avoid cancer. Indeed, it has been demonstrated that a 7-day fast once a year can be used to completely remove cancer cells from the body.

Part of what makes autophagy so powerful is that it operates on a molecular and cellular level, and can even be used to reshape tissues. This aspect of autophagy - that it works on a minute level to efface great changes - may give the discussion of autophagy the impression of a broken record, but it pervades all aspects of the autophagy picture. For instance, fasting and high-intensity interval training (or HIIT) can so dramatically improve health because the minute changes that they cause can lead to large "macro" effects on the body's organs and systems.

Like other health and fitness buzz words, autophagy is used enough that it what it actually means can become obscured. In the first chapter, the reader will be provided with a working definition of autophagy, one that begins to explore the different types of autophagy (which will be examined further in later chapters). The reader will also partake in a discussion on why autophagy works, which will help to draw a thick dividing line between autophagy, apoptosis, and the general concept of cell death.

The benefits of autophagy are extensive enough that books can be (and have been) written on the subject. Indeed, it has been argued that the longevity that we see in certain parts of the world like Japan and Greece can actually be attributed to foods and eating regimens that stimulate autophagy in various ways. It seems to be the case that these areas of the long, continuous settlement have preserved secrets from the very distant past. The major benefits of autophagy include anti-cancer and anti-aging effects, but as the reader has already seen, the benefits do not end there. These benefits will be explored in the second chapter.

The question of how autophagy works is another area upon which books have been written. There are many subtopics within that subject alone. Indeed, this is an area that continues to receive research funding internationally as more is learned about the many ways non-programmed cell death can be stimulated or halted. Cancer cells can prevent the human body from accomplishing apoptosis or autophagy while stimulating autophagy with food, drugs, or dieting can fight cancer and confer other advantages. This note underlies the discussion of how autophagy works, and all of this will be detailed in the third chapter.

There are many ways to stimulate autophagy, some of which the reader will already be familiar with. Intermittent fasting is a popular type of eating regime that has found many supporters in the health and fitness community. Intermittent fasting can allow the man or woman trying it to remove fat while preserving muscle. It does this by actually tapping into how human beings consume food and fast naturally.

Indeed, many modern men and women in the Western world take for granted the wide availability of food that characterizes most Western countries. Your ancestor's thousands of years ago did not have refrigerators, freezers, and pantries to store food year-round so that they might eat at all hours of the day. They would rise early in the morning to hunt and fish, and then they would have to skin and cook their quarry, which meant that they may not eat until noontime or later. This meant that they would have been fasting from their last meal the day before until they were able to eat the meal that they had just prepared. As groundbreaking and powerful as intermittent fasting is, it merely represents a more natural state of living for human beings. Fasting and other ways to stimulate autophagy will be explored in the fourth chapter.

These other methods of stimulating autophagy include water fasting and other prolonged fasting diets.

Extended water fasting has become a powerful way for many men and women to incorporate autophagy stimulation into their daily lives. Although some regard extended water fasting as difficult, the benefits that it can lead to by stimulating autophagy are clear. Diets that involve stimulating ketosis (the creation of ketone bodies) in the body will also be examined along with water fasting in the fifth chapter.

Among the most powerful cohorts of supporters of Autophagy as a process men and women can incorporate into their lives are the health and fitness community. Men and women bodybuilders and fitness enthusiasts can all find ways to incorporate autophagy into their lives as a way of losing fat and preserving muscle. Intermittent fasting is the most obvious way of accomplishing this. Intermittent fasting is generally divided into two types: alternate-day fasting and time-restricted feeding. In the sixth chapter, we will explore how diets that involve autophagy, such as intermittent fasting, can be incorporated into your workout regimen to improve your results.

As we have seen, autophagy can be rapidly and reliably stimulated with food. When one is dieting, it is easy to get into the mindset that food equals bad, but this is not necessarily true. Indeed, this is a type of thinking that must be broken if you truly want to benefit from Autophagy. Most people know that oatmeal first thing in the morning can raise metabolism and lead to fat loss. Well, many foods do basically the same thing but through autophagy. The many foods that can stimulate autophagy will be explored in the seventh chapter.

Fasting is the best way to stimulate autophagy because this period of fast encourages the body to work toward recycling components and improving homeostasis. Most programs that stimulate autophagy involve fasting of some form of another, including the limited type of fasting known as intermittent fasting. But there are other diets that tap into the importance of fasting without actually fasting. The fasting-mimicking diet is just such a diet, and it will be explored along with related topics in fasting in the eighth chapter.

Autophagy is technical enough that most people do not truly understand it and a few dedicate their careers to studying it. In the ninth chapter, the reader will learn tips to help them with stimulating autophagy through fasting. Some want help in fasting for days and days, while others want tips on how to get the most from intermittent fasting. All of the fasting tips you need to get started on your forays into fasting will be explored in the ninth chapter.

Stimulating autophagy is complex, but that does not mean that you and others like you cannot do it. Indeed, it can be said that the autophagy processes are complex, but the stimulation that you can do externally is easy. It may be as simple as not eating for eighteen hours or drinking more water than usual. In the tenth chapter, you will learn how you can stimulate and optimize autophagy by incorporating autophagy secrets and tips into your life.

Autophagy is not a mere fad. Autophagy has been shown to reduce the risk of cancer and lengthen life. Indeed, if autophagy were a drug it would probably be too expensive for you to afford it. Fortunately for you, autophagy is not a drug. It is something that your body does naturally, but which process has been undermined by the Western tendency to overeat and introduce toxic chemicals into the body. *Autophagy: Discover How to Live Healthy and Longer with Your Self-Cleansing Body's Natural Intelligence* will help you to reverse this trend in your own life and improve your quality of life. It all begins with an in-depth exploration of what autophagy is and why it is.

Chapter 1: Understanding Autophagy

Health regimens that tap into the human body's natural methods of achieving homeostasis have become more popular in recent decades as men and women of divergent backgrounds attempt to connect with Mother Nature and all of her secrets. Diets like the Paleo Diet and Atkins all purport to represent more natural ways of eating and living, suppositions that are not always far from the truth. Indeed, assertions made by those who promote these diets, that our ancestors consumed foods high in proteins, fats, and fibers, but low in carbohydrates, these assertions have been supported by the historical record and by scientific discoveries about the body.

Much of the science surrounding Autophagy is based around just this approach: attempting to understand the body's natural way of recycling components and achieving equilibrium. In fact, autophagy can be understood as to how the body naturally achieves a balance between all of its and its needs. The necessity of this type of balance should be clear. Just as a large town or even a business requires a records department, police department, sanitation department, and the like, so too does the human body have to approach its functions from the standpoint of achieving a balance between often disparate goals and requirements.

Just as a large town has a need to remove redundant or unnecessary components, so too does a human body or even a cell. In fact, autophagy occurs at a cellular level: a process that is able to achieve macro or organism-level effects by building on the individual cell and tissue effects that begin often with a simple signal. Autophagy and other processes similar to it are stimulated by various factors that often compete with one another to lead to a result. If the factors in favor of autophagy outweigh those that are against it, than autophagy wins and the body begins to engage in a process that can lead to a number of benefits, which include weight loss, increased energy, the release of human growth hormone, anti-cancer effects, and anti-aging effects.

If the factors discouraging autophagy outweigh those activating or stimulating it, then autophagy is blocked on the cellular level. This often is the case in cancer, where cancer cells are able to release signaling molecules that phosphorylate or otherwise inhibit important protein or signaling molecules. Of course, this mechanism of cancer is not natural to our bodies but represents a dysfunctional error that can lead to death if doctors are not able to treat it. Fortunately, science has a solution here. By finding ways to stimulate autophagy, even in the context of cancer, we can often slow or even reverse the effects of cancer, which can lead to survival.

Studies of the genetics of autophagy are regarded as significant enough that they lead to an awarding of a Nobel Prize in 2016 to a Japanese scientist. Autophagy (and the dysfunctional cancer pathways that interfere with it) is coordinated by an intricate mélange of genes, proteins, signaling molecules, and competing pathways. Of course, this is the norm in the human body, allowing the body to achieve homeostasis by sort of a majority rules decision. As chaotic as it may seem, these types of pathways evolved because they work. Autophagy exists in us because it serves a purpose and does some good.

Autophagy, a type of non-apoptotic cell death, involves the consumption of cellular components by organelles as a result of a signaling pathway. Many different proteins and molecules play a role here, but the more important ones have been well-studied. Indeed, scientists now know enough about these molecules that they can research foods that stimulate them and determine whether claims about health benefits related to these foods have any basis in fact.

The results may come as a surprise to some. It has been shown that foods that activate or stimulate the important AMP-activated protein kinase (which itself stimulates autophagy) have been shown to reduce the risk of cancer, fight cancer, increase longevity, and confer a host of other positive health benefits. This dispels the beliefs of some that diets that purport to tap into more ancient ways of living (like Autophagy) are not based in science or are tantamount to wishful thinking.

Autophagy, the process of using the body's natural cellular autophagy process to confer health benefits, is anything but wishful thinking. In fact, autophagy is occurring in your body right now, and it most likely is acting to preserve your cells (and your body as a whole) from components that would eventually derail it. Think of autophagy as a natural and healthy type of recycling that occurs in your body. This healthy recycling is very far removed from those distorted beliefs about fasting and diet that some detractors spew. Learning more about autophagy, including gaining an in-depth understanding of what it is, may help in your attempts to incorporate this powerful tool into your daily life.

Autophagy Defined

Autophagy, or non-programmed cell death, is a process that is constantly occurring in cells and tissues in the body. Apoptosis occurs at the cellular level, which means that it takes place within the cell membrane through the action of several cell organelles, of which among the most important is arguably the autophagosome. This organelle fuses with the lysosome in autophagy. Autophagy can be defined as the process of cellular breakdown or recycling that occurs within the cell. Some also add to this definition that autophagy processes are able to use components broken down for fuel (hence recycling) with the help of the mitochondria.

The autophagosomes, lysosomes, endoplasmic reticula, mitochondria, and numerous other vesicles and smaller particles within the cell participate in autophagy. Autophagy stems from a Greek root and it means "self-eating." Many in the health and fitness community like to think of autophagy as the breakdown of no longer needed cellular components for energy, which is different from the programmed death or "suicide" of cells in apoptosis. Autophagy occurs on an as-needed basis as opposed to being pre-programmed like apoptosis. This allows autophagy to be upregulated or downregulated as needed, so there will always be cells undergoing autophagy somewhere.

The idea is to upregulate autophagy for the purposes of health and fitness benefits, which are often referred to as Autophagy. Metabolism is important in autophagy as your basal metabolic rate works in tandem with processes like autophagy to cause you to lose weight, maintain the same weight, or to perhaps gain weight. This all happens at the cellular level through the breakdown of components like fat particles in hepatic cells and other body tissues. Autophagy is capable of acting in cells of many different types in the body, which is how it is able to achieve the Autophagy results that most of you desire.

Indeed, autophagy even plays a role in upregulating T1 and T2 helper lymphocytes leading to a stronger immune response.

Autophagy is significant in helping the body fight disease processes and increasing longevity to such a degree that cancer cells attempt to disrupt the process as part of their disordered growth. But we are jumping the gun a little bit. Let us dive deeper into understanding how autophagy works at the cellular level.

Autophagy basically involves different types of phagocytosis that occur within the cell. Phagocytosis is another word that comes from the Greek, and it basically means "cell eating." This word refers to the ability of cells to consume components, generally those that originate outside the cell. As you will soon see, autophagy, although it takes place within the cell, can involve the digestion of components that came from outside of the cell (such as a recycled cell whose components need to be broken down). These components, such as amino acids, can be used to build new components or for energy.

Autophagy can be quite complex, which is why an entire chapter in this book is devoted to understanding how this process works. This process is carefully controlled by signaling processes in the body, but it can be stimulated (and manipulated) by things that we do, such as the activities we do with our body and what we put into our body.

Why Autophagy Works

Autophagy works because the body needs a way of breaking down its own components and using them as material for other cells and tissues, and for energy. Therefore, autophagy represents a way that nature has solved the problem of not generating waste that ultimately serves no purpose. Think about it this way, as human beings, we generate a ton of garbage that is tossed into garbage dumps, sewage sites, and perhaps ultimately makes its way into waterways and oceans. This is trash that serves no purpose after its original purpose is done as it is no longer being used for anything. What autophagy does is take in the body's garbage and recycle it so that only the things the body absolutely needs to get rid of are removed in the renal system and GI tract.

But autophagy is more than a mere way for the body to hold on to its recycling goodies. This process also allows the body to achieve a measure of homeostasis. Homeostasis is a fancy way of saying equilibrium, and all animals must maintain internal and external homeostasis or else they would become extinct. Autophagy is also a way for the body to produce those compounds or molecules that it needs, which is why this process is upregulated in periods of fasting or intense exercise, such as in high-intensity interval training (or HIIT).

This latter type of autophagy is the primary subject of this book. Here we will attempt to understand how men and women can use fasting, exercise, and food to tap into the body's own recycling system. This can allow you to achieve a host of goals, whether they are weight loss, increased immune function, anti-aging benefits, or anti-cancer benefits. The benefits of autophagy are numerous. They will be explored further in a later chapter, but we can introduce some of the functions of autophagy here by way of an introduction. Some of the roles that autophagy plays in the body include:

- Cell death
- Tumor suppression
- Repair of damaged cellular components
- Removal of infectious particles

Autophagy, unfortunately, is also a target for processes that seek to derail it, as we mentioned earlier. Autophagy experiences interference by infectious agents like bacterial proteins and viral particles. Autophagy is also interfered with by tumor cells, perhaps the most well-known type of interference. Tumor cells evolve ways to resist destruction by autophagy and apoptosis, and this often involves the synthesis of proteins and enzymes that interrupt the normal signaling pathway of autophagy. Some of these pathways will be explored in greater detail later.

Autophagy for Health

Most people reading this book are interested in the uses of autophagy for health benefits. You may have learned about autophagy on the internet or on social media, and you are interested in learning more. Some of the claims made about autophagy may seem outlandish. It has been purported that autophagy can have anti-cancer effects, anti-aging effects, and can boost the immune system. It has even been said that autophagy can increase human growth hormone release in the body and cause drastic weight loss. All of these claims are true.

Indeed, scientists have only tapped the iceberg when it comes to all of the powerful things that autophagy can do in the human body. It has been demonstrated that men and women living in places where they consume foods that stimulate autophagy like green tea, ginger, and other foods have been blessed with greater longevity, lower rates of cancer, and other indications of good health compared to other populations. Much study has been devoted to uncovering the secrets of these peoples, and one of the links in the chain may be autophagy.

Autophagy, as you have learned, is a natural body process that helps the human body in several caretaking activities, but it does much more than this. Some of the more significant effects and qualities of autophagy will be explored later, but for now, we can point out some of the more significant aspects. Benefits of autophagy include:

- Ability to fight cancer
- Ability to protect against neurodegenerative diseases, such as Parkinson's Disease

- Ability to regulate other cell organelles to enhance cellular function
- Ability to protect against misfolded proteins that can cause amyloid diseases
- Ability to improve neuroplasticity, brain function, and brain structure
- Ability to strengthen the immune system both directly and indirectly
- Enhancing the growth of cardiovascular cells
- Protecting against aging
- Protecting DNA from degradation
- Protecting the body's organs and tissues from damage

Autophagy is able to accomplish this through the numerous autophagy genes that lead to the release of proteins, enzymes, and signaling molecules that regulate autophagy and other cellular processes in a positive way. The awarding of a Nobel Prize to Yoshinori Ohsumi in 2016 was related to his study of autophagy-related genes, of which there are known to be at least 32. The study of these genes has allowed scientists to elucidate some of the mechanisms of autophagy.

Types of Autophagy (and Induction)

Several different types of autophagy are known, of which microautophagy, macroautophagy, and chaperone-mediated autophagy are the most important. The differences between these three will be explored later, but they will be summarized here. Macroautophagy is regarded as the main autophagy pathway. It involves the eradication of damaged proteins or organelles' using what is known as an autophagosome. Autophagosomes fuse with the more well-known lysosome, which is then able to breakdown, the components.

Microautophagy involves the engulfment of particles by the lysosome directly, without the mediation of the autophagosome. This process generally occurs by invagination, or folding in, of the lysosome's membrane. Chaperone-mediated autophagy is the third major pathway, and it is still being actively studied. This pathway involves the formation of a protein complex and an intricate pattern of recognition. This process is distinct from other types of autophagy because of the specificity that is involved in stimulating it compared to the other types of autophagy.

Autophagy can be induced or stimulated in a variety of ways, all of which will be examined closely in this book. Fasting is one of the most reliable ways of stimulating autophagy, and it is recommended by health enthusiasts who have actively studied the best ways to activate this pathway. Fasting can take a variety of forms, including the well-known intermittent fasting, or so-called alternate day fasting, which involves punctuating days of fasting with "normal" days of eating. Dieting and exercise can also be used to predictably stimulate autophagy. The main ways of stimulating this pathway (that will be examined here) include:

- Fasting
- Dieting with the Ketogenic Diet (or similar regimens)
- Exercise, especially HIIT (high-intensity interval training)

In subsequent chapters, ways in which autophagy can be induced to help you achieve your health goals will be more closely examined. These goals may include weight loss, targeted fat loss, and increase in muscle mass and definition, but they may also include anti-aging benefits and cancer-protective effects. Indeed, many people who decide to fast do it not because they are attempting to align their appearance with their desired body image but because they are interested in living a long, healthy life. It is not necessary to isolate a single goal when it comes to integrating autophagy into your life. There is no wrong goal. Autophagy can help you change your life and your health dramatically, including ways that you may not have been expecting.

Chapter 2: The Benefits of Autophagy

The benefits of autophagy are numerous enough that scientists are still engaged in elucidating them. To some, the benefits of this process are obvious as populations who live a life free from modern processed foods chocked full of chemicals and who are engaged in more physical activity than the average Westerner appear to be blessed with better health and longer lives than others. In this chapter, we will explore the major benefits of autophagy. The purpose of this discussion is not only to help you understand why you should consider ways that you can stimulate autophagy but also help you understand how much you have been missing by not thinking focusing on this important pathway.

You were introduced to the benefits of autophagy in the first chapter. These benefits include:

- Anti-aging capability
- Cancer-fighting ability
- Protection against neurodegenerative diseases, such as Parkinson's Disease
- Regulation of other cell organelles to enhance cellular function

- Protection against misfolded proteins that can cause amyloid diseases
- Improved neuroplasticity, brain function, and brain structure
- Strengthening of the immune system (directly and indirectly)
- Enhancement of the growth of heart cells
- Protecting DNA from degradation
- Protecting the body's organs and tissues from damage

These benefits will be explored in greater detail in this chapter; focusing on the major ways that autophagy can change lives.

Autophagy Can Help with Weight Loss (and Fat Loss)

Autophagy can lead to fat loss through its action in hepatic cells and other areas where fat is stored. The breakdown of fat is termed lipolysis, which literally means "breaking of fat (particles)." One of the remarkable aspects of autophagy is that it occurs in all cell types in the human body, so anywhere you have fat that is damaging to your body or unneeded autophagy can help you mobilize it. The best ways to achieve weight loss and fat loss with autophagy is through fasting, although exercise also works very well. This is why intermittent fasting combined with workout regimens like high-intensity interval training, or HIIT, has been found to lead to dramatic benefits in men and women regardless of the lifestyle of background.

Autophagy Can Improve Your Skin

Our skin is our largest organ. Many men and women do not think of their skin this way, but they should as it allows them to consider all the damage this organ takes from the sun, from chemicals, and from other factors in our environment. Autophagy is designed to help us undo some of the damage that we receive as a result of factors in our body as well as external factors like the sun. Harmful free radicals and other natural and unnatural elements in our environment need to be removed by the body, and autophagy is one of the major ways our body accomplishes this. Fasting, dieting, and exercise can give our skin a healthy glow and this is all thanks to autophagy.

Autophagy Can Improve Digestion

It is important for the cells of your digestive tract to be able to repair themselves and clear junk and other damaging particles. The cells of your mouth, esophagus, stomach, intestines, and other adjacent organs are all tasked with an important function, and that is to help your body process what it takes in and use those components for health. But in the process, your body exposes itself to things that can harm it. This makes autophagy particularly important in the GI tract as this organ (like the skin) is constantly being placed in harm's way. Finding ways to stimulate autophagy in your body can help you regulate your GI tract, leading to improved digestion and overall improved health.

Autophagy Can Improve Exercise Performance

Exercise performance tends to be improved when we engage in activities that activate our body's natural way of behaving. This is part of the reason why skipping breakfast before your morning workout, or even eating a light meal instead of gorging on fast food can make such a big difference. Our bodies are not expecting to be inundated with calories (especially not carbohydrates) early in the morning or before the activity so this tends to make us unregulated and less homeostatic because our body is forced to devote energy expenditure towards food breakdown instead of physical activity. Engaging in physical activity alone or combined with dieting and fasting stimulates autophagy and actually increases our exercise tolerance. This is partly due to more efficient use of energy.

Autophagy Can Prevent Cancer

Autophagy plays an essential role not only in removing damaging (or damaged) components from cells but in removing cells that are dysfunctional or should not be allowed to survive because they are not beneficial to the body. This is where the survival of the fittest analogy comes into play. Just as animals fight for survival in their environments, so too must cell fight for survival with the fewer fit cells being the ones to be removed.

Autophagy not only removes damaging components, but it removes cells that are not fit to stick around. It does this outside the specific programming of apoptosis, targeting cells that are normal enough but not quite fit. By doing this, autophagy can remove cells that have become cancerous or even before they reach this stage. This is part of the reason why cancer cells attempt to disrupt autophagy, a topic that will be discussed in greater detail later. By stimulating autophagy, you are not only strengthening your body's adaptive defenses, but you are helping to undo the deceptive tactics of cancer cells.

Autophagy Can Boost the Immune System

Autophagy has been shown to boost the actions of T1 and T2 helper cells. Autophagy has also been shown to stimulate other aspects of immune function and to play a role in the regulation of inflammation. Inflammation can occur as a result of trauma or injury, or it can be part of the immune system's response to infection. Stimulating autophagy can, therefore, protect you from infection as well as give you a healthier balance in times of inflammation. This means that inflammation can be localized to areas where it is needed, preventing you from feeling sicker than you need to be while your body is hard at work in clearing whatever ails it.

Autophagy Can Reduce the Risk of Neurodegenerative Diseases

Autophagy has neuroprotective effects, which means it can protect you from developing Parkinson's Disease, Alzheimer's

Disease, and other forms of dementia. This type of benefit is similar to some of the other benefits that have been mentioned on this list, as it is a function of the ability of this natural process to improve cellular function and longevity by helping it to remove poor components and recycle. Neurodegenerative diseases can be the result of a natural process of aging or they can be due to damage from free radicals, misfolded proteins, or other forms of stress. Just as you cannot prevent yourself from aging, you also cannot fully prevent yourself from being exposed to damaging particles. By stimulating autophagy, you are able to strengthen your body's natural way of protection, regardless of where your body's damage is coming from.

Autophagy Can Improve Your Metabolism

Autophagy is involved in lipolysis and other aspects of energy production. Indeed, autophagy is capable of using many of the components that it recycles for energy with the assistance of cell organelles, such as the lysosome, endoplasmic reticula, and lysosome. Stimulating autophagy is able to improve your metabolism by shifting your body in favor of recycling and energy production rather than energy storage in the form of fat cells or adipose tissue. Part of this picture also has to do with the ability of autophagy to improve insulin sensitivity.

Insulin insensitivity is the hallmark of type 2 diabetes, a condition characterized by continuously elevated levels of insulin in the bloodstream leading to the body developing resistance to insulin. High levels of insulin are in turn related to the body constantly being exposed to high levels of sugar in the blood. This means that stimulating autophagy by dieting and fasting is particularly beneficial, although exercise also can be useful here too. This improvement of metabolism – your body's breakdown of components as part of a healthy basal metabolic rate – has dramatic long term benefits regardless of what your goals are with autophagy.

Autophagy Can Improve Your Quality of Life

It has been demonstrated that stimulating autophagy can lead to men and women to feel subjectively healthier and more energetic. Part of this has to do with the ability of stimulation of this pathway to help with anxiety, depression, and other issues of mental health, but there are also aspects of autophagy that lead to wellbeing, a finding that is not entirely understood. Although science has identified dozens of autophagy genes, it is likely that the number of genes, proteins, and factors that play a role here will increase over time as this process because better understood. The improved sense of wellbeing, energy, and general health may be related to the CNS benefits that were discussed previously or they may be something different entirely. Studies suggest that how you stimulate autophagy is no important here, so exercise, fasting, dieting, or all three can be useful here.

Autophagy Can Lengthen Your Life

The anti-aging benefits of autophagy are a hotbed of research and discussion, and it is not difficult to understand why. Human beings have long searched for a miracle drug that can lengthen life and improve health, and it may turn out that that miracle drug is a process that our bodies have been engaging in since we were born. Autophagy is a natural way that our body protects us from damaging particles, infectious agents, and cancers. This process is also part of our normal process of recycling its components and using them to build other things and for energy.

As confusing as it may sound, autophagy has also been demonstrated to have anti-apoptotic effects. In other words, autophagy can extend life by discouraging apoptosis. By helping the body to achieve homeostasis and remove damaging particles, autophagy can prevent the activation of apoptosis triggers. Conversely, prolonged autophagy can actually stimulate apoptosis. The takeaway point here is that autophagy is designed to help us, and by stimulating it consistently and well we place ourselves on track for lives that are long, healthy, and filled with all of the other benefits of autophagy that were mentioned here.

Some of the benefits of autophagy actually involved multiple different specific benefits working together to create an overarching benefit, as is the case in anti-aging. As you have seen, autophagy actually causes anti-aging effects through several different mechanisms. Anti-aging can result from improved metabolism and cell turnover, or it can be a result of protection from neurodegenerative disease and cancer. Some aspects of anti-aging were not detailed here, including protection of DNA from damage. One way that autophagy protects DNA is through its protection from free radicals. These free radicals can shorten telomere and lead to DNA errors. Stimulating autophagy, therefore, can lead to greater telomere length, which indirectly increases longevity, a finding which some have informally labeled the telomere effect.

Other benefits of autophagy that have not been mentioned include the ability of this process to protect specific types of cells from damage or to improve them in dramatic ways, as is the case with the cells of the heart. The benefit of improvement in cardiovascular function through the action on heart cells is obvious, as the heart is an organ whose dysfunction is closely associated with morbidity. A particular area that will be touched on in this book is the ability of autophagy to aid men and women in achieving their specific health and fitness goals.

An understanding of what autophagy is and why it is beneficial is merely a precursor to a detailed explanation of why autophagy works. Most readers would not be motivated to dive into the gross details of autophagy without first getting a crash course on why autophagy is important. We have been exposed to the three main types of autophagy (macroautophagy, microautophagy, and chaperone-mediated autophagy) and a true understanding of this subject requires a more detailed examination of these subjects. In chapter three, you will gain more detail on the different types of autophagy and what they mean for you.

Chapter 3: How Autophagy Works

Autophagy exists because it works. Autophagy is a way that our body can repair damaged tissues or components without having to resort to apoptosis. Apoptosis should be thought of as a last resort. Programmed cell death is what our body must turn to when its components are absolutely beyond salvation. But sometimes cells and tissues are capable of being repaired and recycled. Indeed, sometimes the problem is an individual cell or an individual protein. If the body can merely get rid of this bad component then it cannot only restore its function, but it can improve it by removing a weak link in the chain. When we remember that these broken down components are then used to build new ones, the underlying benefits of this process to a complex organism like a human being becomes obvious.

In this chapter, we will examine how autophagy works by exploring the three major types of autophagy, namely macroautophagy, microautophagy, or chaperone-mediated autophagy (or CMA). These types of autophagy frequently work together to achieve the desired metabolic or exercise effect, but occasionally they have individual roles, as is the case of the role of microautophagy in helping the cardiovascular system deal with the drug rapamycin. Understanding the different types is the beginning of understanding in more detail the complexity of autophagy and how this complexity can really be distilled into three simple tools: fasting, dieting, and exercise.

The three main types of autophagy discussed here generally involve the operation of well-known cellular organelles, such as the lysosomes, endoplasmic reticulum, ribosomes, and mitochondria, although lesser-known structures such as the autophagosome and phagophore will also be discussed. As with other chapters in this book, some aspects of detailed terminology are explained in the glossary for reference purposes. The reason for exploring this subject is not to inundate the reader with details, but to help them make connections that may be of use to them later when it comes to being better understanding.

The Basics

Autophagy is a housekeeping tool that involves several organelles working together to accomplish the goal of keeping the cellular house in order. This may mean removing components that are damaging to the cell-like free radicals, processing degradation products so they can be reused for energy or repurposed, and even deciding that the cell itself should be degraded because it no longer meets the needs of the organism (in this case, the human body). The basic unit of autophagy function has been traditionally regarded as the lysosome, but further studies in recent decades have revealed that this organelle takes a back seat to a structure called the autophagosome.

This is not to say that the lysosome is not important. This organelle is extremely important, both in terms of the autophagy process and in related pathways like apoptosis. The lysosome is a double membrane structure that contains enzymes and other protein complexes that are capable of degradation and signaling. This allows the lysosome to work alone for breakdown, although it typically works in concert with other organelles. The name of the lysosome literally means "breaking (or breakdown) body."

The lysosome receives components for a breakdown from a double membrane vesicle known as the autophagosome. The presence of a double membrane is important as it allows components from outside the cell to be introduced into the interior of the cell, and it also allows the autophagosome to fuse with the lysosome, which contains enzymes and other necessary components. The movement of the autophagosome to the lysosome for breakdown and recycling occurs via the movement of microtubules which pull the organelles this way or that. This is the basic foundation for most autophagy pathways.

Macroautophagy

Macroautophagy is a process that utilizes several steps to trap components in the cytoplasm and recycle them. The first step is the formation of a structure called the isolation membrane. The formation of this structure is triggered by specific factors, some of which will be discussed further shortly. This structure is formed within the cell's cytoplasm; that is, the "sea" of fluid within the cell, as opposed to extracellular fluid outside the cell membrane. Cells are very good at using membranes to separate extracellular components from intracellular ones. This is a means of regulating what is able to enter the cell and protecting the cell.

The second step after the formation of the isolation membrane is the formation of a structure known as the phagophore: a larger structure compared to the initial isolation membrane. The phagophore undergoes a process of expansion which leads to the engulfing of components in the cytoplasm and the formation of a third structure, the autophagosome. The autophagosome may be thought of as the basic essential structure of autophagy. This structure moves towards an important organelle called the lysosome, which results in the fusing of the autophagosome with the lysosome. The result is that the contents of the autophagosome are dumped into the lumen of the lysosome for degradation and recycling.

As it would be against the interests of our bodies to be degrading components willy nilly, macroautophagy is controlled in a highly nuanced manner by a series of triggers. Many of these triggers are in turn signaled and regulated by a number of proteins encoded in genes. Autophagy-related genes, or Atg, refer to proteins involved in the steps that lead to the formation of the autophagosome (via elongation).

Triggers of macroautophagy (in general terms) include:

- Fasting or starvation
- Lack of oxygen in the lungs
- Presence of reactive oxygen species
- Presence of infectious agents
- Therapeutic agents or drugs (like chemotherapy)

Microautophagy

In macroautophagy, the lysosome passively receives the vesicle (the autophagosome) containing the components intended for degradation and recycling. The autophagosome fuses with the lysosome in this case. In microautophagy, the lysosome is the main actor, directly engulfing the components in the cytosol that are intended for degradation. This process involves the double membrane of the lysosome folding in around the components that are being brought into the organelle, a process known as invagination. Like macroautophagy, this process is stimulated by specific triggers, of which factors in the environment are known to be significant.

Chaperone-mediated Autophagy (CMA)

Chaperone-mediated autophagy, or CMA, is an interesting pathway that is an active area of research. This type of autophagy also relies on the lysosome. In this pathway, particles designated for destruction are tagged with a molecule known as a chaperone. The chaperone is there to tag along, alerting the cell's organelles (particularly the lysosome), that this article is intended for destruction. The particle with the chaperone is recognized by receptors on the lysosomal membrane, which then invaginates the particle.

Other Types of Autophagy

There are several other types of autophagy that have been studied. Some of these fall under the three categories of macroautophagy, microautophagy, and chaperone-mediated autophagy, while others can be regarded as standalone pathways. For example, aggrephagy is regarded as a type of macroautophagy. Some lesser-known types of autophagy include.

Zymography: the detection and degradation of granules in the pancreas

Xenography: the degradation of toxic and infectious particles

Ribophagy: the breakdown of ribosomes

Pexography: the breakdown of peroxisomes (a type of organelle)

Mitophagy: the breakdown of mitochondria by lysosomes

Lipophagy: degradation of lipid droplets by autophagy

Chlorography: the protection from sunburn in some organisms

Aggrephagy: the degradation of cellular protein aggregates in macroautophagy

Autophagy Use in Therapeutic Agents

Autophagy has garnered attention in recent years for a number of reasons, not least of which is the potential use of autophagy as a target of therapeutic agents. That autophagy can be targeted for use by therapies for a wide number of purposes should come as a surprise to no one. Autophagy has already proven itself to be a tool that can be useful in cancer, weight loss, infection, and inflammation. In particular, autophagy has received attention for its potential uses in cancer.

Cancer therapies are often highly damaging to the person undergoing them. Chemotherapy and radiation can damage normal cells right alongside the abnormal ones, forcing scientists to find ways to streamline these sorts of therapies in order to spare normal tissue as much as possible. But therapies based on autophagy work by different means, and they have the potential of doing very little harm to non-cancerous cell. This is a function of autophagy's role as an entirely normal cellular process in human beings, which places this pathway in juxtaposition to chemotherapy and radiation which are essentially toxic therapies designed to be used against cancerous cells.

There are two main roles that therapeutic agents that operate based on autophagy can play in cancer. The first role is the use of therapeutic agents that attempt to stimulate autophagy and remove cancerous or otherwise dysfunction cells. In this scenario, a drug would stimulate autophagy in a particular cell type (like hepatic cells, for example), which would lead to the body naturally clearing cancerous cells and their components in the liver. The second role may be a little counterintuitive to some. This second role would involve therapeutic agents to block autophagy and trigger apoptosis in the cell.

Blocking autophagy may seem like something that you would not want to do, but in the case of cancer cells, there is a reason to take this route. Autophagy is also used to preserve cells that may be damaged or exposed to damaging particles, like infectious particles or free radicals. Autophagy does not only remove malfunctioning cells, but it saves those cells that can and should be salvaged. By inhibiting autophagy in cancer cells, the body will be able to trigger apoptosis in these cells and clear them, which would theoretically result in the clearing of a cancerous tumor. Indeed, cancer cells have evolved numerous ways of preserving themselves using genes and one of these ways is to prevent apoptosis from being triggered in cancerous cells.

Recall the apoptosis is programmed cell death, and it can be triggered by a number of factors and thresholds in the cell. Essentially, these triggers are designed to lead to cell death when it is clear that the cell has passed a threshold where it can (or should) be salvaged. The body is able to recognize that rapidly replicating or otherwise dysfunctional cells like cancerous tumors are "bad" and should be removed by the body using apoptosis. The cancer cells block apoptosis, causing these cells to be preserved when they should not be. By blocking autophagy in these cells, therapeutic agents can push the balance in favor of apoptosis.

Naturally, understanding autophagy deeply requires an in-depth understanding of how it can be stimulated or encouraged. Now that you understand the benefits of autophagy and the major pathways through which it operates you can begin to explore the major ways to stimulate this important process. In the next chapter, you will learn more about the three major mechanisms by which you can encourage autophagy in your body and reap all of the benefits.

Chapter 4: Stimulating Autophagy

When it comes to the benefits of autophagy, most people know about fasting. Indeed, fasting is so powerful a tool in humans that religious and spiritual groups the world over have incorporated fasting into their calendar of holy days and practices. But fasting is not the only way to stimulate autophagy. Indeed, specialists have come up with ways of mimicking fasting in order to trick the body into thinking it is fasting, allowing men and women who wish to benefit from fasting to partake of those benefits without having to deal with the downsides that usually come along with it.

Of course, most people choose to go about fasting the old fashion way; that is, to actually stop consuming calories. And the process of fasting is not as straightforward as some people like to think. For example, what should you drink when during a fast? Is it okay to consume decaffeinated products? What should you eat before you start fast? Your body's digestive process and other functions can be modified by fasting so what should you eat when breaking a fast? These questions and many others are perfectly legitimate ones, and they reveal that there is more to autophagy than most people think.

In fact, there is more to autophagy than you think. Autophagy is how your body incorporates Darwinian principles into its daily operations. In other words, autophagy is a type of survival of the fittest on a cellular level. Your body would not be a well-oiled machine if it was highly wasteful in its operations. For this reason, your body has learned to recycle components that it has consumed because it was weak, including not only components within the cell, but cells and tissues themselves.

The purpose of this is to make the body better. It is a selfish process that allows cells to survive because they are more suited to the purposes that the body needs them for. This allows the body itself to be better at surviving compared to other "bodies" (which is why the process involved in the first place). This is all part of a larger homeostatic process. The human body is constantly engaged in a balancing game of breaking things down and building them up. This breaking down and the building is balanced in order to achieve the homeostasis the body needs to survive as long as it can.

A good example of this is the bone. The bone has cells in its marrow called osteoblasts and osteoclasts. Osteoblasts are the cells responsible for laying new bone, while osteoclasts are the cells responsible for breaking down bone. Now it may seem as if breaking down bone may be a bad thing. It is if this breaking down is not balanced with building up bone, as is the case in osteoporosis. The reverse situation is also true. Building up too much bone can be bad as it can lead to bones that abnormally think and less functional than our body needs to be.

The normal situation (and the desired one) is for the body to be constantly breaking down and building up the bone to a certain degree in order to maintain bone homeostasis. This equilibrium allows the bone to be remodeled in response to stress. So if you ride horses a lot, the osteoclasts break down your bone while the osteoblasts reform bone that will take a slightly different shape in response to the stress of the horse's back against the long bones of your legs. The result is the bow-leggedness that we associate with cowboys and other prolonged riders of horses.

Stimulating autophagy is therefore about tapping into this type of homeostasis. It is not an all or nothing equation, which is typical for the human body (i.e. non-all-or-nothing situations). Life on Earth is about balance and even life in your body is about a measure of balance. Your goal, therefore, is to tap into this balance and shift the scale in favor of those things that encourage the sorts of things that you want. Let us jog our memories and recall what some of the reasons for wanting to stimulate autophagy are. The reasons why you want to activate or stimulate autophagy include:

- Greater weight loss or fat loss
- Improved metabolism and insulin sensitivity
- Improved immune functioning
- Improved DNA repair and stabilization

- Anti-aging effects
- Anti-cancer effects
- Improved exercise tolerance
- Improved cardiovascular function
- Improved nervous system functioning
- Protection from neurodegenerative disease
- Protection from infection
- Improved sense of health and wellness
- Improved quality of life

These are the sorts of things that most men and women would want. There are few people living today who would admit to wanting a short life filled with cardiovascular disease, neurodegenerative disease, poor DNA stability, and insulin resistance. Regardless of what your specific goals are, there is certainly a role played by autophagy as a constantly occurring process in the achievement of your goals. In this chapter, we will review the three main ways that you can stimulate autophagy in order to improve your goals.

But before we do that, let us spend a moment thinking about what stimulating or activating autophagy means. All it really refers to is shifting the equilibrium balance in favor of autophagy as opposed to maintenance of poor cellular and tissue function and eventually apoptosis. Recall that apoptosis is programmed cell death, and this happens when your body is not able to salvage a cell because it is old, poorly functioning or damaged. Your goal is to encourage autophagy rather than apoptosis because the former is associated with improved health outcomes and longevity while the latter is not.

It is also important to remember that autophagy is stimulated by general environmental or contextual factors, specific environmental changes, and specific enzymes and proteins related to the first two states. So starvation and fasting are general environmental (for the body) factors that encourage autophagy while drinking green tea gives you specific chemicals that also stimulate autophagy without actually causing an "environmental" factor change in the body. Many of these triggers of autophagy involved an important protein called AMP-activated kinase, which is responsible for stimulating autophagy on a molecular level.

So what are the major ways of stimulating autophagy? These should not come as a complete surprise. They are listed below:

- Fasting
- Dieting
- Exercise

Under the scope of dieting, we include intermittent fasting and extended water fasting, which will be covered in more detail in this book. Under the heading of dieting, we include eating regimens like the well-known Ketogenic diet, which involves consuming a diet very low in carbohydrates or no carbs at all.

Related diets include the Atkins diet and the Paleo diet. Exercise is a means of stimulating autophagy that is often ignored, though, as we have seen it is an important trigger because of its ability to improve metabolism and other processes closely tied to autophagy.

Fasting

Fasting is regarded as the best way to stimulate autophagy. Although different studies have different recommendations regarding how long you can fast, some in the industry argue that a single 18-hour fast can be enough to kill cancer cells in the body. Others have recommended longer periods of fasting, such as a day-long fast, with days of more regular eating before and after. It is interesting to ponder whether the incorporation of fasting rites into religious practices actually represents a way that early modern humans managed to incorporate their observations about health and longevity into their religious practices and taboos.

Fasting essentially is a period in which you deprive your body of calories of any kind. Fasting stimulates the release of factors that activate autophagy, like AMP-activated kinase. These periods of fasting have numerous benefits aside from just losing weight, although even this is mediated by autophagy which is involved in the process of lipolysis (the breakdown of fat or adipose tissue). Many men and women fear to fast because of misconceptions they have about it. Fasting does not have to be for a prolonged period. Indeed, the most popular type of fasting in the health and fitness community is intermittent fasting, which involves incorporating hours without eating into your daily eating schedule (which will be discussed in more detail later).

Dieting

Dieting is also able to stimulate autophagy by similar means to fasting. Although fasting is regarded as the gold standard when it comes to stimulation of this important pathway, many men and women are able to achieve very dramatic results with dieting because it also taps into the same metabolic and tissue breakdown pathways as fasting (although in a less dramatic fashion).

This is an opportune time to talk about the Ketogenic diet, which will be discussed at length in a later chapter. The Ketogenic diet is designed to place the body in ketosis, which involves the release of molecules called ketone bodies from the liver. Ketosis has been associated with a wide variety of health benefits, almost as many as autophagy. The big problem with ketosis is that prolonged ketosis can be damaging to the body, and some medical conditions render ketosis life-threatening because of morbidity concerns (as in type 2 diabetes).

There is a lot of misinformation out there about the Ketogenic diet. The Ketogenic diet has become very popular very quickly because of the dramatic effect it can have on changing your body. Many men and women have gone from obesity to a normal BMI with Keto. The benefits of the Ketogenic diet include:

- Reduction in blood glucose
- Increase in insulin sensitivity (and reduced insulin levels)
- Improved organ functioning
- Improved concentration
- Lower triglyceride levels
- Lower blood pressure
- Lower blood sugar

Exercise

Exercise is a stimulator of autophagy that is easy to overlook. Many people attempt dieting and exercise and do not lose weight (a common goal), which is why they often look askance at programs that focus on these two things. But an exercise regimen that is consistent and involves a measure of muscle strain and cardiovascular activity can dramatically benefit the body in ways outside of the desired weight loss or muscle building. Indeed, many people fall prey to adopting a workout program that does not place enough emphasis on intensity. Your goal in your exercise program should be to get your heart rate up. It is this stress on the body that leads the body to change itself in ways that benefit you.

Much attention has been paid lately to HIIT, or high-intensity interval training. A program of HIIT cannot only dramatically change your body's appearance but increase aerobic and anaerobic capacity. That is, the ability to tolerate exercise in cases where your muscles have adequate oxygen, and in cases where they do not. HIIT and other types of exercise increase the rate of autophagy, which improves exercise tolerance, improves concentration, and increases the rate of fat breakdown (or lipolysis).

A question that is important to ask is how much HIIT is too much. It is important to remember that HIIT is meant to be done in intervals, which means that not all of your workouts (or sets within a workout) or at the same high level of intensity. Not only does prolonged high intensity weaken your muscles and increase the risk of injury, but prolonged high intensity can actually lead to apoptosis, which is certainly something that you want. You can think of this as another case where equilibrium or homeostasis is coming into play.

Muscle growth is the result of muscle breakdown which forces the muscle to grow. In other words, when you are working out intensely, you are stressing and breaking down muscle fibers, which force them to become hypertrophied so that they can better handle stress in the future. You want to shift the balance in favor of slightly increased breakdown so that during periods of rest you can have greater repair. This is an example of using your body's normal equilibrium in the right way. But if you were to be too intense in your training, you would be causing an overwhelming shift towards breakdown, not allowing your body to recover, which leads to permanent injuries (like muscle tears) and apoptosis.

Studies of moderate exercise and high-intensity interval training have shown differences that are based on autophagy. Both exercise programs cause an improvement in immune functioning, and of course can cause things like weight loss and improved body image, but there are powerful results specifically associated with HIIT. These results are consistent with what we would expect from an exercise program that is specifically using autophagy to impact the body during exercise. These benefits include:

- Better aerobic metabolism
- Better aerobic performance
- Better pulmonary ventilation
- Better peak VO2 (volume of oxygen)

Chapter 5: Water Fasting and Ketosis Diets

One of the advantages of autophagy as a solution to your health problems or goals is that it can be stimulated in various ways, as we have seen. We have discussed fasting at length as a trigger for autophagy in the human body, and we will discuss exercise (in addition to intermittent fasting) in the next chapter. The purpose of this chapter is to explore some of the major ways that dieting can be used to stimulate autophagy: one of the body's major pathways that can lead to targeted fat loss.

There is a thin line between a fast and a diet. Most fasts discussed in this book are really diets that involve periods of fasting. This is particularly true of intermittent fasting, which has become one of the most popular ways to lose fat and preserve muscle in the health and fitness community. If you are thinking that dieting versus fasting is really a matter of semantics than you are right. Most fasting is really dieting because if you were to fast forever than that would actually be starvation. Most people who "fast" on purpose intend to break that fast, which means they have to put some thought into such things as what to eat before the fast and how to break the fast (i.e. what to eat afterward). In this chapter, we focus on dieting, specifically two diets whose effects are closely linked to autophagy: extended water fasting and ketosis diets.

Ketosis diets are really an umbrella term for diets that seek to achieve just that: ketosis. Ketosis is the state of ketone body production in your bodies. Ketone bodies are normally produced from fat mobilized in the liver in response to starvation. Ketosis can sometimes be a bad thing, as is the case with type I diabetics who present to the emergency room in Ketogenic shock. But ketosis is also associated with positive states in the body, which has led to ketosis being used for weight loss and a host of other health benefits. In this chapter, we deal specifically with the Ketogenic diet, although other diets like the Atkins Diet also operate via ketosis.

Extended Water Fasting

Water fasting uses nutrient deprivation to trigger autophagy in the body. Water is an essential element for human survival, but it does not contain any calories and cannot be used for energy. This means that you can drink as much water as you want and still be in starvation as far as the body is concerned because you have not taken in any products that can be used for energy. Ultimately, this is what the body uses "food" for: as a source of energy and other essential nutrients and building blocks the body requires.

A water fasting diet is, therefore, a diet that involves supplanting meals with water in order to maintain the body in a fast for a prolonged period. In this regard, a water fasting diet is not too different from an intermittent fasting diet, which will be discussed shortly (in the next chapter). Intermittent fasting involves separating periods of eating by periods of fasting, which can take up a whole day or just part of a day. This can also be done on a water fasting diet.

Your water fasting diet can take up a portion of your day or it can last for 1-2 days. A longer fast with water is known as an extended water fasting diet, and some people choose to fast this way for 7 days or longer. Seven days is a big number as studies have shown that this number of days is enough to completely remove cancerous cells from your body (if you are in a precancerous state). This is because cancer cells are rapidly dividing and cannot survive without nutrients over this period of time.

Your water fasting can take any form that you would like it to. Naturally, you will have to make sure that you are drinking adequate quantities of water or you will really find yourself in trouble. Diets like this work because during this period of fast your body is using autophagy for lipolysis and other metabolic processes that lead to weight loss. Some people feel that water helps them to feel full, which is why water diets can be effective rather than a dry fast. Choose the duration of water fasting that works for you, making sure to be start off slow and be realistic with your expectations or risk backsliding into your poor eating habits.

The Ketogenic Diet

The Ketogenic diet is probably the best known of several diets that operate by triggering ketosis. Ketosis is a period of altered body functioning that is triggered by the presence of ketone bodies in the bloodstream. Indeed, ketosis merely means the state of having ketones in the blood. There are three ketone bodies whose production is triggered by prolonged periods of starvation or fasting. The three ketone bodies produced during ketogenesis are acetoacetate, beta-hydroxybutyrate, and acetone. Although prolonged ketosis can be harmful and even fatal, there are positive benefits that are seen in ketosis. Some of these overlap with the benefits of intermittent fasting and autophagy in general.

Ketosis is triggered by a state of extremely low carbohydrates. For this reason, the Ketogenic diet and other diets that operate based on ketosis like Atkins have their clients consume diets extremely low in carbohydrates. Carbs are considered bad because they increase your circulating glucose concentration and cause major problems with insulin sensitivity and metabolism. At the practical level, the body stores excess sugar as fat, which is not what are most people going on a diet want?

In the Ketogenic diet, an eating program high in fat and protein is consumed. Fat and protein do not cause problems with metabolism and insulin so they are not problematic in this protocol. Also, the idea is to replace carbs with other sources of calories, and these are the two other macronutrients that the body can resort to for energy. Ketogenic diets are very low in carbohydrates. Less than 10% of total daily calories are consumed from carbohydrates. So if your caloric intake should be 2000 calories for the day, this means that you would only be consuming 200 calories from carbohydrates, which is about 50 grams. That is less than one 16 oz. bottle of soda. Most people on Keto consume even fewer carbs, i.e. 100 calories or 25 grams of carbohydrates.

It is important to be realistic when starting any diet. This means determining that a diet fits in with any health problems you have. But it also means thinking about whether you will be able to stick to the diet and perhaps what things you need to do before starting the diet. Keto is not for everyone, but those who have tried it and reaped the benefits swear by it.

Chapter 6: Autophagy for Muscle Mass

Autophagy is just as useful for preserving muscle as it is at for losing weight. This is part of what makes autophagy-dependent programs a lifestyle rather than merely a diet. In stimulating autophagy through fasting, dieting, or exercise you create a new paradigm for your body that triggers a series of changes that leads to an entirely new health outlook. Men and women who experience fatigue, a weakened immune system, and obesity can suddenly find that they are losing weight, more energetic, and less prone to colds than they had formerly been. And all of this is due to finding ways of incorporating autophagy stimulation into their lives.

As you have already seen, activating autophagy is as simple as remembering three simple words: dieting, fasting, and exercise. We can also add a fourth word – food – but technically this is part of dieting. Food will be explored further in the next chapter as it is a simple and reliable way to stimulate autophagy. Dieting and food also allow you to improve your metabolism, which will not only lead you to look better and feel better but to have more energy and longevity. Some even describe a glow that people have because of autophagy. This is not pseudoscience.

Autophagy has been shown to provide benefits to skin, hair, and other organs: all as a result of the improved functioning of the body that results from careful and considerate stimulation of this process.

Some of you may be wondering what autophagy can possibly have to do with working out and muscle mass. It has everything to do with it, to be honest. Autophagy improves your metabolism, increases your insulin sensitivity, and burns fat, through direct lipolysis. These are all things that men and women interested in building muscle, or merely in looking better and losing weight, hope to achieve. Stimulation of autophagy pathways is essential to anyone looking to improve their bodies by adding muscle without having to resort to illicit performance-enhancing drugs.

Intermittent Fasting

This is a convenient juncture to begin the discussion of intermittent fasting, one of the most popular diets in the health and fitness industry right now. Indeed, intermittent fasting is popular even outside the fitness industry as many men and women have discovered how this diet can dramatically alter their bodies and their lives. Intermittent fasting has the term fasting in it, but it really out to be thought of as a type of diet. This is because, in intermittent fasting, one of the most important things that the dieter needs to do is to learn to pay attention to macronutrients as well as total caloric intake.

Indeed, it is a myth in both the Ketogenic diet and intermittent fasting that the total amount of calories consumed is unimportant. Although some people who consume high caloric diets as part of their sport – like professional athletes, bodybuilders, and powerlifters – might pay less attention their calories than others would this does not mean they are unimportant. In intermittent fasting, it is important to pay attention to the total number of calories consumed in a day and when you are consuming them as part of keeping track of your macronutrients (or macros) and in order to make sure that you are eating enough in order to meet your respective macro needs for the day.

In other words, in intermittent fasting, you have to pay attention to calories or risk finding yourself hungry because you did not properly estimate how much you need to eat during your eating window. This brings us to a discussion of what precisely intermittent fasting is and how it works. Intermittent fasting is essentially what it sounds like. It is a diet (or eating program) that involves a period of fasting separated by periods of eating. The duration of the fasting period can vary based on the specific regimen adopted by the dieter. Intermittent fasting is usually divided into two types:

- Alternate-day fasting
- Time-restricted eating

These are similar. They only differ in terms of whether the fasting lasts for an entire day or part of the day. In alternate-day fasting, the dieter spends an entire day (24 hours) without eating, while in time-restricted feeding the day is divided into periods of eating and fasting. Both alternate-day fasting and time-restricted feeding are popular ways of going about this diet with men and women finding ways of making the eating schedule work in their often hectic lives.

Time-restricted feeding, however, has received more attention from the health and fitness media because it has attracted a number of influential supporters in the community. This type of diet is popular for bodybuilders and fitness competitors who are looking to shed fat and preserve as much muscle as possible. Although calories are important and need to be planned carefully, this type of diet can allow you to consume high calories as long as they are within a certain window.

So how does the time-restricted feeding type of intermittent fasting diet work? It is pretty simple. The dieter comes up with a particular window in hours that they will be allowed to eat in the day and fasts for the rest of the day. A popular type is the so-called 16/8 split. This protocol involves consuming all of your meals in an 8-hour window and fasting for the remaining 16 hours. This would take the form of eating, say, between 11AM and 7PM (an 8-hour window) and fasting the rest of the day. This split has been shown to be very effective at shedding fat, but you can use whatever window you choose. It can be a 20/4 window, in which you only eat for four hours in the day, or it can be more or less restrictive.

Intermittent fasting brings with it all of the benefits of autophagy that have been discussed in other areas of this book. It also has some benefits of its own. These have been elucidated by vigorous study both inside the fitness community and outside of it. The benefits of intermittent fasting are numerous. Here are some of them:

- Improved fat loss
- Improved cardiovascular functioning
- Improved glucose control
- Increased lifespan
- Reduced muscle loss
- Reduced hunger
- Improved metabolism
- Improved self-image and energy
- Reduced risk of cancer
- Reduced risk of neurodegenerative disease

Incorporating Intermittent Fasting into Your Workout Plan

If you have an active workout regimen (or an active life), it is important to choose a diet that works with your workout and other responsibilities. Fasting is difficult for many people because they feel they need the calories that come from food for their occupation, their workout regimen, or just for the energy to get them through a day filled with screaming children or obnoxious bosses and coworkers. There is nothing wrong with that. Intermittent fasting can allow you to have shorter periods of "fasting" in your day so you are able to eat as you need.

The key is to come up with a schedule that fits with your life. For example, if you need to be at work at 8AM and you typically go to the gym at 6AM, perhaps you should consider a 16/8 intermittent fasting split with an eating window between 7:30AM and 3:30PM. This will allow you to squeeze your eating period into your busy day. For those whose obligations are later in the day, you may want to push your eating window back a little so that you are not engaging in heavy activities on an empty stomach.

Little side notes about eating before a workout: many fitness enthusiasts have found advantages to working out on an empty stomach. Although your energy levels may be slightly reduced at first because you are used to having sugar constantly in your bloodstream, it has been shown that working out on an empty stomach increases your metabolism, improves insulin sensitivity, and provides a host of other benefits. Consider working out on an empty stomach if you work out first thing in the morning. You could always have your first meal in your window after your workout.

Other things to keep in mind here will be touched on in the Frequently Asked Questions section. Some are curious about what they should eat before a fast, after a fast, or whether it is safe for them to fast. These questions and many more will be answered. All you have to do is keep reading.

Chapter 7: Foods that Stimulate Autophagy

Most of you reading this book are likely doing so not because you plan on writing a paper and submitting it to a journal. Most likely you have a specific goal that you plan to achieve with Autophagy and you are looking for tools to help you achieve that goal. Your goal may be weight loss, it may reduction in cancer risk, or it may just be feeling better through dieting or fasting. If any of these are your goals, thinking about the sorts of food you should eat is clearly something that would be beneficial to you.

In this chapter, we will review some of the major foods that have been shown to stimulate autophagy. We will choose several foods to explore in detail. Naturally, all of the foods that play a role in stimulating autophagy cannot be examined in detail because if they were, you would find yourself reading a book solely about that. So what are the foods that you can incorporate into your diet in order to stimulate autophagy? Some of the major foods in this category include:

- Ginger
- Green tea
- Reishi mushrooms
- Turmeric/curcumin

These foods each stimulate autophagy although they do it in different ways. Some readers may notice that several foods on this list are regarded as superfoods that provide a wide host of benefits. These are foods that are consumed in some traditional cuisines, especially in East Asia and South Asia. These are areas where residents most likely identified early on that these superfoods provided benefits for health and longevity, even if they may not have understood why exactly in these early days.

You may be asking yourself how you can incorporate these foods into your diets. Some of these, like green tea, are easily incorporated. Drinking one to two glasses of green tea in the first half of your day is not difficult to do. It might be a better idea to drink tea in the first portion of your day because the caffeine in your tea can keep you up at night. There are also are some particular aspects of green tea to keep in mind (which will be explored shortly). Ginger and Reishi mushrooms are ingredients that can be conveniently added to a wide variety of dishes, such as salads or soups. Turmeric/curcumin is a dry spice that also can be added to meat dishes or a wide variety of other dishes. Getting a benefit from these does not require that you go overboard, although if you find that you like one or more of these and would like to add more to your mealtimes, it is generally safe to do this in the case of the four foods provided here.

Ginger

Ginger is one of those foods that are so good for you that it is difficult to overstate its power. Indeed, ginger has been shown to have dramatic anti-oxidant benefits that place it as a great resource for those dealing with an infection. Ginger has also been purported to increase longevity. This last claim should come as no surprise as research has shown that ginger directly stimulates autophagy, which will be explained further shortly. Ginger exists in the form of a thick and fragrant root. It has a characteristic odor and taste. Ginger together with honey is a traditional and very effective remedy for resolving the common cold.

For our purposes, it is important to note that ginger contains a number of important compounds. These include gingerol as well as a group of compounds known as shogaols. 6-shogoal is the most common of this group of chemicals. These chemicals are similar in structure to gingerol. 6-shogaol is believed to be the more important compound in autophagy. It has been shown to induce autophagy in cancer cells, but not programmed cell death (apoptosis). This has been shown to be particularly powerful in lung cancers. Incorporating ginger in your diet will help you boost your immune system and fight off cancer, all through the power of autophagy.

Green Tea

Many volumes have been written about tea and its benefit. Here, we focus on one of these teas: green tea. Green tea is a popular variety although it does compete for sales with some of the other varieties. Indeed green tea is just one of many different commercially available teas that have been demonstrated to provide health benefits to those who drink it. Green tea also has antioxidant properties and is believed to have anti-aging benefits. It boosts autophagy in the skin and can improve organ function, too. In fact, one should keep in mind that even if particular foods are associated with particular benefits, because they stimulate autophagy they are likely to provide some of the other autophagy benefits too (like improved metabolism) even if it is to a slightly lesser degree.

The compound that we are interested in is called EGCG. Epigallocatechin gallate, or EGCG, is a catechin found in teas. EGCG has a polyphenol structure and it is the most abundant catechin found in tea. Also contained in other foods, EGCG has been studied extensively because of its many potential health benefits. EGCG stimulates autophagy in hepatic cells leading to lipolysis, or lipid breakdown. EGCG accomplishes this by increasing the concentration of AMP-activated protein kinase. As we have seen, AMPK is a direct stimulator of autophagy

Reishi Mushrooms

Mushrooms can easily be added to many different meals. Reishi mushrooms would break a fast although it is worth it because of its autophagy benefits. Adding Reishi mushrooms to your diet has been shown to reduce the incidence of colon cancer. Reishi mushrooms do not demonstrate their effects through AMP Kinase, but through another pathway called the mitogen pathway. Reishi mushrooms have also been shown to have a role in stabilizing the nervous system. Adding this mushroom to your diet really can go a long way in helping you feel better and experience positive health outcomes.

Turmeric/curcumin

Turmeric/curcumin is a spice that is commonly found in South Asian cuisine. Indeed, in some parts of India turmeric is put in most dishes. Curcumin in turmeric does not have the best bioavailability, but this can be increased by consuming black pepper along with this orange/brown spice. Turmeric is a component of Indian Ayurvedic Medicine as are the other items in this list of autophagy stimulators. Turmeric specifically is regarded as having great neuroprotective effects and anti-inflammatory powers. Turmeric also plays an anti-cancer role through the mediation of AMPK (activating it through phosphorylation). Adding turmeric to your intermittent fasting or Ketogenic diet dishes can go a long way in further boosting the autophagy benefits you already expect.

Chapter 8: Stimulating Autophagy by Mimicking Fasting

Imitating fasting with the so-called Fasting Mimicking Diet is an option for men and women who would like the benefits of fasting, but may have reasons why fasting is not the best choice for them. Fasting is regarded as the gold standard in terms of stimulating autophagy because of its demonstrated use in triggering the body to remove damaged, poorly functioning, or dysfunctional components, such as cancer cells. But autophagy can also be stimulated well by diet and exercise, and in the case of the Fasting Mimicking Diet, the goal is to create a diet that resembles fasting without actually being fasting.

Recall that the idea behind fasting is that it replicates how our human ancestors would have eaten tens of thousands of years ago. At this time, human beings would have lived primarily as hunter-gatherers and not in the settled agricultural societies that characterize the way nearly all humans on Earth live today. This means that humans would not have had access to storehouses filled with grain, sugar cane, processed foods, and all the other goodies that many people take for granted today. If you wanted to eat, you would have had to hunt or fish your quarry or risk starvation.

Now, this type of life may seem harsh, but our bodies adapted to survive in this type of environmental context. It is not too different from how apex predators like lions and tigers live in their environments today. They spend much of their day sleeping or guarding their territory (essentially a fasting period), while they devote a portion of their day to hunting and eating. Naturally, when a lion hunts he's or she is generally obeying both a predatory urge and a physical urge. He or she is hungry. This means that the fasting period actually serves to motivate the lion to hunt and hunt well. You rarely see obese or out of shape lions because their way of life demands that they are a well-oiled machine.

Well, human beings were once not too different from these apex predators. We also used to spend much of our days sleeping or guarding are territories, and we would have hunted on an empty stomach. Obesity would have been rare in social groups where food was not instantly available and men and women would have had to hunt for survival. Today, we are constantly exposed to food in frankly enormous quantities, including high concentrations of sugar that would have baffled our ancestor. What some diets do is focus on what we take into our body as a way of preventing the lowered metabolism and energy drain that comes from eating diets high in carbohydrates.

The Fasting Mimicking Diet allows men and women who are interested in reaping the benefits of diets like the Ketogenic diet or intermittent fasting to tap into those benefits without all of the restrictions. The Fasting Mimicking Diet involves devoting five days out of a 30-day period to caloric restriction similar to what is seen in Keto while the remaining 25 days are less restrictive. The idea here is to place the body in something akin to ketosis in order to mobilize adipose (fat) stores for energy rather than the circulating blood sugars that most people who eat sugar and carbs constantly use for energy. This excess sugar is not only used for energy but stored as fat which is counterproductive and leads to obesity. By cutting out sugar sources, you force your body to look to other more natural energy sources. This leads to benefits like fat mobilization (lipolysis) through autophagy as well as other benefits like improved insulin sensitivity.

Basics of the Fasting Mimicking Diet

The essential fact to remember about the Fasting Mimicking Diet is that during your five days of the fasting mimicking you are drastically reducing your caloric intake but not actually going on a fast. A fast means that you are not taking in any calories at all, and during your fasting-mimicking days, you would be taking in perhaps as little as 500 calories. Five hundred calories would be equivalent to one large cheeseburger at a fast-food restaurant or a large highly processed pastry (that is high in fat and carbohydrates).

As the Ketogenic diet, what you eat during your fasting-mimicking days is important as the idea is to trick your body into thinking that you are fasting. You do this by eating a diet that is relatively low in carbohydrates, but not as low as it would be in Keto. Recall that the hallmark of Keto is that carb intake is reduced to almost zero. In Fasting Mimicking, you may take in about 30% of your calories from carbohydrates. It is okay to do this because your total caloric intake is so low (between 500 to 1000 calories for five days).

The idea here is that this period of low calories is recognized by the body as starvation, which is the essential goal of a fast. Fasting and starvation are distinguished by the body merely by duration. For example, any period of no food is technical "starvation" to the body although we tend to use this term only to refer to periods where individuals have no caloric intake for a prolonged period usually due to circumstances outside of their control. Prolonged starvation can lead to syndromes like kwashiorkor or marasmus that are seen in countries experiencing drought or other calamities.

To return to our main point: tricking your body into thinking that it is in starvation because of days of low calories triggers autophagy. Most people on the Fasting Mimicking Diet do it because they want to lose weight, but all of the other benefits of autophagy can be reaped here, too. This is a recurring theme in this book. Autophagy confers a host of benefits to the person who stimulates it, and you might find that you reap positive health advantages that you had not anticipated, like a sense of energy and well-being.

The main benefit of the Fasting Mimicking Diet is that you can enter something like a fast without some of the downsides of a fast (or starvation). Some people may find fasting difficult because they have never done it before. Others may have health concerns that render fasting inadvisable. The Fasting Mimicking Diet allows you to stimulate autophagy similar to how you would in a fast. Again, research suggests that fasting of 18 to 24 hours is the best way to stimulate autophagy (and reap its benefits), but not everyone can do this. Some people use the Fasting Mimicking Diet as a starting point to attempting fasting in the future.

Example of a Fasting Mimicking Diet Protocol

A typical Fasting Mimicking Diet protocol consists of 5 consecutive days of fasting-mimicking followed by 25 days without fasting mimicking. Most practitioners of this diet carefully follow their macronutrients (macros) just as they would in the Ketogenic diet. Typically the first of the five days is lower on carbohydrates, but the carbs are increased slightly in the following days. There are different ways to go about this diet, but an example of a diet using this protocol is shown below. The percentage shown is the relative percentage of total calories for the day from that macronutrient. Recall that the three main macronutrients are fat, protein, and carbohydrates.

First Day (Day 1):

A total of five to six calories total for each pound of body weight, so about 800 calories for a 160-pound person

Fat: 60%

Protein: 10%

Carbohydrate: 30%

Following Days (Days 2 through 5):

A total of three to four calories in total for each pound of body weight, so about 480 calories for a 160-pound person

Fat: 50%

Protein: 10%

Carbohydrate: 40%

Chapter 9: Tips to Help with Fasting

Some people learn best with tips. Let's face it, there is a lot to learn about autophagy, and no one is expected to be an expert after reading about the subject for an hour or two. You will learn the most about this process after you have given stimulating it a try. Tips can help you whether your goal is to lose weight or too fast for days and days in order to kill cancer cells in your body. Here are some tips to help get you started.

Tip 1. You do not have to skip meals in order to fast.

Although fasting means that you are not eating, it does not necessarily mean that you have to skip a meal. What are we talking about here? People who intermittent fast and have a 16/8 split, for example, are still able to eat a normal (or relatively normal) three meals a day. They just have to do this in a smaller window than they normally might. So your breakfast might be at 10 AM, your lunch might be at 1:30, and your dinner might be at 5:30. Fasting is a different word from "starvation" for a reason. Fasting does not have to mean that you are miserable.

Tip 2. Having coffee before you start your fast (or something else with fat in it) can keep you satiated.

There is a lot of talk about whether or not coffee drinking should be considered breaking a fast. Part of this subject will be discussed in more detail shortly. In truth, there are some calories in coffee, but they are so low (generally less than 100 calories) that they are not counted by many people who fast. But for the purpose of this trip, we are thinking about ways that you can work coffee in before you fast. If you have coffee right before a fast it can help keep you satiated, especially if it contains some cream or other additives with a little added fat in it.

Tip 3. Drinking water during your fast can help you feel fuller.

Water fasting is a thing for a reason. No, not because some people are lunatics who like to drink water until it makes them sick (which is actually a thing). Water can help you feel fuller. There is some debate as to whether this is due to receptors in your stomach being stretched by the volume of water or because of some other reason, but all you need to know is that works. It may not be a good idea to replace all of your next five meals with water when you are just starting out with this, but it is something to keep in mind. Having a tall glass of water can help you stave off your hunger when your goal is to fast for a short while longer.

Tip 4. Work your way up to longer fasts rather than jumping into a long fast early on.

Taking baby steps is always a good idea. When it comes to fasting, this means not jumping into a highly restrictive fast, but working your way up to it. It is not difficult to do. Indeed, some people do this by first engaging in an autophagy diet like intermittent fasting and then working their way up to a whole day fast or longer. Again, you always have the option of drinking water as part of your fast thereby incorporating a water fasting diet. Most people who fast for days and days started out where you might be now - a little overweight and wondering if it is possible to make a major change in their life. The answer is "yes," it is possible.

Tip 5. Eating a pinch of salt during a fast can quench your hunger pangs.

Some fasting experts recommend eating a pinch of salt during periods when you are tempted to break your fast. Salt is sodium chloride, which means it contains two ions that are essential in your body's homeostasis. Sodium chloride not only can satiate your taste buds, but it can help you feel fuller (and better) by keeping the water in your body. Have you noticed that when you drink large quantities of water you tend to urinate it out relatively quickly? That is because your body needs sodium chloride in order to keep the water in your body's cells and tissues. So here is a little trick. If you are having problems with your fast, try adding a pinch of salt.

Tip 6. Apple cider vinegar may break your fast but it will help you while intermittent fasting.

Apple cider vinegar contains acetic acid which assists in vitamin and mineral uptake in the body. The acetic acid in the vinegar will help your body to absorb the vitamins and minerals that your body consumed in foods hours earlier. Apple cider vinegar also contains polyphenols that boost the immune system. Besides that, some people like the taste of apple cider vinegar so consuming this can help you get the most out of what you have eaten earlier so you will not feel as hungry.

It is a matter of debate whether or not apple cider vinegar will break a fast. Some in the health industry argue that it does not contain enough calories to impact insulin so it will not break a fast. Others say that apple cider vinegar is not zero calories, and even one calorie is enough to break a fast. Even if you drink this right before you start a fast you can have a benefit during your fast. To incorporate this type of vinegar into your fasting regimen. You will not regret it.

Tip 7. Adding a pinch of sea salt to your water can help you maintain your fast.

Salt does not have to be a bad thing. We have already spoken about adding a pinch of salt, but it is important here to talk about the benefits of all-natural options during your fast. Processed products, like artificial sweeteners, can actually cause problems with your fast because they can derail your metabolism. Even salt can have other things added to it that make it more than just regular salt. So if you are planning to use salt to help you along in your fast, try sea salt or another of nature's varieties of this substance.

Tip 8. Avoid supplements like branched-chain amino acids during your fast because these will cause an insulin spike.

Whether or not to take supplements is always a big question when it comes to fast. Many people continue to take supplements during their fast without being aware that they are technically breaking their fast because their supplements are not calorie-free. Even branched-chain amino acids (or BCAAS) contain calories, which makes sense considering that some people actually use these for energy during a workout. So here is a tip: it is okay to take supplements and vitamins before or after a fast, but they should generally be avoided during your fasting window. If you do not, then you really are not fasting.

Tip 9. Do not add creams or sweeteners to drinks you are consuming during your fast (such as coffee); you also should not use artificial sweeteners like those contained in diet sodas.

Tip 10. Tea will not break a fast so drink lots of green tea (which will cause you to feel satiated).

Tea is another one of those products that have tons of questions surrounding it when it comes to fasting. Does tea break your fast? Although some choose to avoid tea and anything else substantive like this during a fast, many fitness experts argue that tea will not break your fast. They argue this because tea does not contain compounds that impact metabolism (specifically, it does not impact insulin causing an insulin spike) so you can drink as much tea as you like and your body will still think you are fasting. Green tea can also help you to feel satiated while you are on your fast.

Chapter 10: Tips to Help You Optimize Autophagy

There are many tips out there that can help you to optimize autophagy and achieve your health and fitness goals. Some of these are things you can do while other tips are items that may help you to keep in mind. Here is a free one: food is not necessarily a bad thing. Eating food will cause you to break a fast as your body has to metabolize that food (which sets off a whole chain of metabolic events), but food can do good things for you two. This food fallacy that says that *all* food is *always* bad: well, this is an idea that you should get out of your thinking as quickly as you can. Below are some other tips that can help you make the most out of your dieting, exercising, and fasting with autophagy.

Tip 1. Educate yourself about autophagy.

The best first thing you can do is to educate yourself on the subject. Rome was not built in a day, and your ideal body and perfect life will not be built in a day (if they ever will be built at all). What you need to do is to learn the most about autophagy so that you can know how to do the rights things and avoid the wrong things. If you have read this far then you have already taken an important step in that direction. Here is an opportunity for us to push you on towards continuing that journey.

Tip 2. Ease your way into your new lifestyle.

One of the worst things you can do in any dieting or exercise regimen is to be overambitious. This is not to say that ambition is bad - it certainly is not – but being too ambitious can lead you to be a little unrealistic about what you can accomplish early on in your dieting adventure. If you are used to eating more than 2000 calories a day and consuming lots of sugary drinks as well as other sources of carbohydrates then it will be quite an adjustment for you to do fasting, intermittent fasting, ketogenic diet, or even exercise programs like those involving HIIT. The best thing you can do for yourself is to ease your way slowly into your new lifestyle rather than jump in headfirst.

Tip 3. Incorporate autophagy-stimulating foods into your fasts and diets.

There is a reason why an entire chapter of *Autophagy: Discover How to Live Healthy and Longer with Your Self-Cleansing Body's Natural Intelligence* is devoted to foods that you can eat. Food is one of the best ways that you can stimulate autophagy because everyone needs to eat. You may even find that you like the sorts of foods that are part of your new dieting regimen.

Tip 4. Make a habit of calculating the calories in your foods.

This one is a biggie. Some men and women are already in the habit of tracking the calories in all the foods that they eat. For others, this is a practice that seems unrealistic: one that they will never be able to incorporate into their lives. Keep in mind that you need to start somewhere. If you do not keep track of calories already, you can start by making a habit of reading the labels on all of the foods that you purchase. Those labels are there for a reason. When you realize how unhealthy some of the food that you eat is you may find that you no longer have a desire to eat it (and that is often a good thing).

Tip 5. Make a habit of paying attention to the macronutrient composition of your foods.

Once you have started reading labels you can begin to understand what they mean. The labels on your food not only tell you how many calories are in your food, but they break down your calories by macronutrients. Proteins and carbohydrates have four calories per gram of weight while fat has nine calories per gram. This is why fat slows down your digestion. Your labels also give you a general idea of how much of each macronutrient you should get in the day and how much that particular food is giving you out of that total. These recommendations from the FDA are pretty liberal, but understanding them is an early step in getting the most out of autophagy.

Tip 6. Start eating healthier (less processed) foods.

Once you have started to feel the changes that come from fasting, dieting, and exercise you will be motivated to make other changes in your life. Although this book has not spent a lot of time talking about processed foods, one of the goals of *Autophagy: Discover How to Live Healthy and Longer with Your Self-Cleansing Body's Natural Intelligence* is to help you realize how the things you do are tied to your body's underlying (and natural processes). Most of you will be motivated to continue being healthy and eating less processed food is a huge step in the right direction in terms of bettering your metabolism.

Tip 7. Start buying foods from farmer's markets and local sellers rather than bigger chains.

For some people, the question becomes how you can begin to eat healthier when it feels like everything around you is unhealthy. If you recognize this situation, then you are being very perceptive. Most people in the Western world are inundated with toxic food choices and many people do not have the willpower to resist the temptation to eat unhealthily. An easy way to fix this problem is to surround yourself with healthy food, like those found at your local farmer's market.

Tip 8. Incorporate food timing into your dieting, fasting, and exercise schemes.

Food timing is big in the health and fitness industry. One of the most obvious examples of this is the popularity of oatmeal. Many in the industry advise eating oatmeal in the morning. The reason for this is that oatmeal is a type of complex carb that increases your metabolism. A high metabolism puts your body in fat-burning mode throughout the day. As a slow metabolism is common in obesity-plagued populations, like those in the United States, paying attention to food content and timing can be an easy way to get the most out of autophagy.

Tip 9. Be realistic about what you will and will not be able to accomplish on a diet.

Diets fail for a number of reasons, but one of the big ones is that dieters are not realistic about their diets. In other words, a new dieter will plan to eat 500 calories a day for five days not realizing how little this is in terms of food and that it is unlikely they will stick to this diet. Be realistic. Perhaps you can start at 1000 or 1500 calories a day and work your way to 500 (or whatever your particular dieting goal is).

Tip 10. Combine exercise, fasting, and dieting to help you optimize results.

The best way to optimize autophagy is to combine the three main mechanisms of this pathway into one new lifestyle. Instead of deciding whether or not you want to fast, exercise, or diet, how about you do all three? This is not a hard thing to do. An intermittent fasting diet that involves exercising multiple times a week will accomplish all of this for you.

Glossary

6-Shogoal - the most common of a group of chemicals found in ginger known as shogaols. These chemicals are similar in structure to gingerol. 6-shogaol has been shown to induce autophagy in cancer cells, but not apoptotic cell death.

AMP Kinase - AMP-activated protein kinase is an important enzyme that plays multiple roles in the body, including fatty acid absorption, glucose activation, and oxidation. These processes are part of the larger homeostasis or equilibrium that must be maintained in the body both on a macro level and on a molecular level. AMP-activated protein kinase is sometimes referred to as AMP Kinase or abbreviated as AMPK. AMP Kinase is important in autophagy, and many of the stimulators of autophagy involve activation or increasing concentration of AMP Kinase.

Apoptosis - pre-programmed cell death. Apoptosis is believed to be regulated by a series of triggers or thresholds that stimulate cells and tissues to initiate the process of cell death. Apoptosis, or programmed cell death, should be distinguished from non-programmed (or non-apoptotic) cell death, of which the most pressing example is autophagy.

Atg - autophagy-related genes, of which at least 32 are known.

ATP - Adenosine triphosphate, or ATP, is the major energy molecule found in human beings and most other animals. ATP also plays an important role in homeostasis because of the effect that its breakdown and components have in body tissues like the muscles and liver.

Autophagy - a type of non-apoptotic cell death that is regulated by a variety of genes, proteins, and signaling molecules. The name originates from the Greek and it refers to "self-eating." Autophagy is part of the body's normal process of removing components that are superfluous or non-functional, which makes it distinct from the programmed cell death of apoptosis. Autophagy occurs on a cellular and molecular level through the work of proteins, enzymes, and cellular organelles such as the lysosome.

Cell Death - the general name for the process of destruction of a cell or cellular components. Cell death in the human body is usually divided into apoptotic and non-apoptotic cell death. Autophagy is a type of non-apoptotic cell death, which indicates that though it is carefully regulated it is not programmed in the same manner that apoptosis is.

Chaperone-mediated Autophagy - In this pathway, particles designated for destruction are tagged with a molecule known as a chaperone. The chaperone is there to tag along, alerting the cell's organelles (particularly the lysosome), that this particle is intended for destruction. The particle with the chaperone is recognized by receptors on the lysosomal membrane, which then invaginates the chaperone-tagged particle.

Dry Fasting - the informal name for fasting that is not water fasting.

EGCG - Epigallocatechin gallate, or EGCG, is a catechin found in teas. It is a polyphenol and the most abundant catechin found in tea. Also found in other foods, EGCG has been actively researched because of its potential health benefits. It stimulates autophagy in hepatic cells leading to lipid breakdown. It accomplishes this by increasing the concentration of AMP-activated protein kinase.

Fasting Mimicking Diet - a diet that involves devoting five days out of a 30-day period to a low carbohydrate diet similar to what is seen in the Ketogenic diet. The idea is to "mimic fasting" by shifting the body into Keto during that period so you would basically reap the benefits of a five-day fast even though you actually were eating. During this period, autophagy is used to mobilize fat in hepatic cells and other fat storage areas.

HGH - human growth hormone. Human growth hormone is important in bone and organ growth, health and vivacity, and anti-aging. Human growth hormone levels can be increased by fasting, but these effects are only seen in longer periods of fasting.

HIIT - High-intensity interval training. High-intensity interval training has been shown to improve autophagy. High-intensity interval training uses autophagy to stimulate lipolysis (burning of fat).

Intermittent Fasting - a dieting regimen that involves incorporating periods of fasting into your eating schedule. The most common form of intermittent fasting today is a time-limited program in which the day is broken up into periods of fasting and periods of eating. The schedule is divided into hours of fasting and hours of eating. For example, a 16/8 schedule would mean 16 hours of fasting in the day and 8 hours of eating. Most intermittent fasters choose an eating window, such as 12 noon to 8 PM, that works with their commitments and allow them to easily keep track of when they should be fasting and when they are allowed to eat.

Ketogenic Diet - a diet that involves consuming foods that are extremely low in carbohydrates (or have none), which leads to the production of ketone bodies in the liver. The three ketone bodies produced in the liver are acetoacetate, beta-hydroxybutyrate, and acetone. These ketone bodies can be broken down into a molecule called acetyl-CoA and used as a food source. Ketone bodies are known for their characteristic smell, which has been described as fruity.

Ketone Bodies - the name for three bodies produced by the liver when the body has entered "ketosis" as a result of fasting, starvation, disease process, or other conditions. The three ketone bodies produced by the liver are acetoacetate, beta-hydroxybutyrate, and acetone. These are broken down into a molecule called acetyl-CoA and used as energy.

Ketosis - the state of production of ketone bodies in the liver that typically results from long periods of food deprivation as occurs in fasting or starvation. Ketosis involves autophagy, and many diets like the Ketogenic diet have the explicit goal of inducing ketosis. Ketosis is controversial because although this state has some health benefits, it also can result in poor health outcomes if prolonged or associated with a serious condition, such as diabetes mellitus.

LDL - low-density lipoprotein.

Lysosome - an organelle in the cell that is involved in autophagy through phagocytosis. This organelle works in tandem with other cell organelles, such as the endoplasmic reticulum and the mitochondria to accomplish breakdown of cellular components both as a part of autophagy and outside of it.

Macroautophagy - a process that operates via several steps to trap components in the cytoplasm and recycle them. The first step is the formation of a structure called the isolation membrane. The formation of this structure is triggered by specific factors, some of which will be discussed further shortly. This structure is formed within the cell's cytoplasm; that is, the "sea" of fluid within the cell, as opposed to extracellular fluid outside the cell membrane. Cells are very good at using membranes to separate extracellular components from intracellular ones. This is a means of regulating what is able to enter the cell and protecting the cell.

The second step after the formation of the isolation membrane is the formation of a structure known as the phagophore: a larger structure compared to the initial isolation membrane. The phagophore undergoes a process of expansion which leads to the engulfing of components in the cytoplasm and the formation of a third structure, the autophagosome. The autophagosome may be thought of as the basic essential structure of autophagy. This structure moves towards an important organelle called the lysosome, which results in the fusing of the autophagosome with the lysosome. The result is that the contents of the autophagosome are dumped into the lumen of the lysosome for degradation and recycling.

Macroautophagy is controlled in a highly nuanced manner by a series of triggers. Many of these triggers are in turn signaled and regulated by a number of proteins encoded in genes. Autophagy-related genes, or Atg, refer to proteins involved in the steps that lead to the formation of the autophagosome (via elongation). Triggers of macroautophagy include fasting or starvation, lack of oxygen in the lungs, presence of reactive oxygen species, presence of infectious agents, and therapeutic agents or drugs.

Microautophagy - In microautophagy, the lysosome is the main actor, directly engulfing the components in the cytosol that are intended for degradation. This process involves the double membrane of the lysosome folding in around the components that are being brought into the organelle, a process known as invagination. Like macroautophagy, this process is stimulated by specific triggers, including various environmental factors

OMAD - one meal a day. Essentially an intermittent fasting diet that involves fasting for 23 hours and eating for one hour a day. Other variations include eating one meal a day every other day, an even longer type of intermittent fasting split.

Phagocytosis - the process of consumption of cell particles, foreign organisms, and debris by lysosomes. Phagocytosis comes from Greek and means "cell eating." It literally refers to the process by which lysosomes, important organelles in the cell, consume and breakdown components with the aid of other organelles, such as the endoplasmic reticulum. This process is generally carefully regulated in the cell with the aid of signaling molecules.

Prebiotic Fiber - foods high in fibers that encourage the growth and maintenance of gut flora. Gut flora is normal bacteria in our GI tract that help us break down food. Examples of prebiotic fiber include artichokes, asparagus, bok choy, and other similar vegetables.

Telomere Effect - the anti-aging effect that can result from fasting. Increasing telomere length can extend the lifetime of our cells and lead to anti-aging benefits.

Water Fasting - an eating regimen that involves supplanting water for food. So the individual will drink quantities of water as part of their fast.

Frequently Asked Questions

1. **What is Autophagy and why is it important?**

    Autophagy refers to the process by which the body degrades and recycles cellular components. Autophagy the term comes from the Greek and it refers to "self-eating." The recycled components can be used as energy. Autophagy can be thought of as a sort of survival of the fittest that occurs on a molecular and cellular level. Cells that are not up to a certain standard are degraded and the components can be used to make new cells. Therefore autophagy can be thought of as important in helping the body achieve a positive balance or homeostasis.

    Autophagy is triggered by a number of set factors, including starvation or fasting, lack of oxygen, and the presence of damaging agents such as infectious particles, reactive oxygen species, and others. Autophagy is a form of non-apoptotic cell death, which means that it is not programmed. This does not mean that autophagy occurs haphazardly. Autophagy is triggered and regulated in a highly nuanced way. Factors that stimulate autophagy are always in play as our factors that inhibit it. This allows the right balance to be stuck in a particular tissue.

2. How can I make autophagy work for me?

Most readers are interested in improving their health in one way or another. Autophagy is a natural process that can be tapped into in order to cause dramatic changes in a completely balanced and healthy way. Some people are interested in weight loss and fat loss while others are interested in prolonging their life or improving their quality of life. Autophagy can be used for weight loss because it is the primary tool for lipolysis (fat breakdown) in hepatic tissue and other areas. This means that the best way for you to mobilize fat is to find ways to stimulate autophagy.

But the uses of autophagy extend far beyond weight loss. Much research in the last two decades has focused on how autophagy can be used in specific ways, like to fight cancer. Scientists are in the process of developing targeted therapies that operate by interacting with the body's pathway of autophagy. Some of these therapies stimulate autophagy while others inhibit them. In the case of cancer, stimulating autophagy can remove cells before they become cancerous. Inhibiting autophagy in cells that are already cancerous can push them into apoptosis.

3. **Is autophagy different from apoptosis? If so, how?**

Apoptosis is programmed cell death. Like autophagy, apoptosis is triggered by a number of factors that the body uses to determine when a cell is no longer needed. In this case, programed just means that once the trigger has been set off, the cell goes through stages of cell death as part of a programmed pathway. Apoptosis is distinct from autophagy in that apoptosis occurs in cells and tissues that cannot be salvaged, and it is associated with death rather than recycling. Apoptosis is almost a self-destruct switch as in a science fiction movie. Autophagy is different. This is a non-programmed cell death that is designed to improve the overall function of the organism.

4. **Is autophagy safe?**

Autophagy is safe because it is a natural process that is constantly occurring in your body. Autophagy allows the body to streamline its cell complement and improve its functioning without having to resort to apoptosis. Autophagy is a process that allows the body to breakdown cells and uses them for energy. In a way, the body feeds on itself in order to be the most ordered, streamline machine that it can be. You should always consult your doctor before beginning any dieting regimen, but you can rest assured that autophagy is entirely safe for you.

Indeed, research has not only found that autophagy is safe but stimulating it is beneficial. The benefits of autophagy are numerous enough that papers detailing them are constantly being published. When it comes to safety, the issues are less of autophagy in general and more concerns about fasting. There are certain medical conditions where fasting can be problematic. Diabetes types 1 and 2 and pregnancy stand out as notable ones. So while autophagy itself is completely safe and natural, some may want to avoid prolonged fasting as a means of stimulating autophagy.

5. Are there any benefits to Autophagy aside from dieting?

Many people who learn about autophagy do so because they are interested in shedding pounds and improving their appearance. But the benefits of autophagy extend far beyond the mere desire to fit into a smaller jean size. Autophagy has been shown to increase longevity, fight cancer, prevent cancer, improve immune function, improve metabolism, improve nervous system functioning, stimulate the release of human growth hormone, and the list goes on. Autophagy is able to do this by having general roles in all cell types, but also by acting in specific ways in specific tissues. For example, autophagy is responsible for the fat breakdown in hepatic cells (lipolysis).

6. Why does autophagy exist?

Autophagy exists because it works. Autophagy is a means for our body to repair damaged tissues, cells, or cellular components without having to resort to programmed cell death or apoptosis. Autophagy is non-programmed or non-apoptotic cell death. Apoptosis should be regarded as a last resort. Programmed cell death is what our body must turn to when its components are beyond the point of salvation. Before this point, some cells and tissues are capable of being repaired and salvaged. In fact, the problem is often an individual cell or an individual protein rather than a damaged area.

The problem may just be that these areas have been exposed to an infectious agent, free radical, or other factors of ultimately external origin. If the body can remove this bad component then it can restore its function and improve it by removing a weak link in the long chain. Remember that these broken down components are then used to build new ones. This should make obvious the underlying benefits of this process to a complicated organism like a human being.

7. Are there different types of autophagy?

There are three major types of autophagy in addition to a large number of subtypes. Autophagy is divided into types based on its mechanism of action. In other words, how autophagy is able to degrade and recycle components. The major types of autophagy are macroautophagy, microautophagy, and chaperone-mediated autophagy (or CMA). Macroautophagy is regarded by some scientists as the most important type. All three involve complex interactions of organelles within the cell.

Macroautophagy occurs via the action of a structure called the autophagosome. This is a double membrane structure that eventually fuses with the lysosome, dumping its contents into it. The autophagosome is formed in stages, beginning with a structure called the isolation membrane. Microautophagy involves primarily the lysosome, which engulfs cellular components by invagination. The third major type of autophagy is chaperone-mediated autophagy. In this type, a molecule marked for degradation is tagged by another molecule called a chaperone. This chaperone is recognized by the lysosome which then degrades the targeted component.

8. **Do I have to fast in order to stimulate autophagy?**

You do not have to fast in order to stimulate autophagy. Indeed, one of the great things about autophagy is that it can be stimulated in several major ways. Indeed, this picture is so nuanced and complex that one can actually make autophagy work better by incorporating all three major ways of triggering autophagy in your life. The three major ways to stimulate autophagy are through fasting, dieting, and exercise.

Fasting is considered the gold standard for autophagy activation. This is because the human body has been designed to operate on occasional periods of fasting, and most of the many benefits of autophagy have been explicitly linked to fasting, The amount of time that is needed to fast is not set with some choosing to fast for less than 16 hours in a day. It has been suggested however that the ideal fast is between 18 to 24 hours (at least). This type of fast has been shown to be effective at clearing cancer cells from the body. But autophagy can also be stimulated well by diet and exercise. Indeed, both intermittent fasting and the Ketogenic diet have been shown to work well with exercise to trigger powerful autophagy.

9. **Is intermittent fasting a "type" of autophagy?**

Intermittent fasting is basically a stimulator of autophagy rather than a "type" of autophagy. Intermittent fasting is interesting because it is both a type of fasting and a type of diet. Intermittent fasting can involve fasting for an entire day or for a portion of the day. Fasting for a portion of the day is known as time-restricted eating or feeding, and it would involve only eating in a particular window, say, an eight-hour period, and then fasting for the rest of the day. Intermittent fasting has been shown to work well with an exercise program, such as a HIIT program, although it can also be used as a standalone trigger for autophagy.

10. **Is it safe to do intermittent fasting or other types of fasting to stimulate autophagy if I am diabetic or have another serious health condition?**

You should always consult a doctor before starting in any health, fitness, or dieting program. This is especially true if you have health problems that require you to take medication. Although human beings have been fasting for hundreds of thousands of years and fasting has been shown to be healthy in most people, there are some cases in which this type of diet may be contraindicated. Many diabetics are able to intermittently fast, but because they have to monitor their blood sugar it may be necessary to either have a generous eating window or to be prepared to break their fast if necessary. Intermittent fasting, however, would certainly be safer than the Ketogenic diet, which would be contraindicated in diabetics.

11. Are there any advantages to intermittent fasting compared to other types of diets that are based on autophagy?

One of the main benefits of intermittent fasting is that, if you do the time-restricted protocol, you are able to incorporate periods of eating into your day rather than fasting for longer periods or even the whole day as you may in other types of diets. This may work better with the schedules of some people. It also works for people that have health problems that making fasting difficult or flat-out contraindicated. There are other benefits to the intermittent fasting diet as well. These have been specifically shown to be found in intermittent fasting although some of these benefits overlap with the overall autophagy benefits. Some of these benefits include improved fat loss, improved cardiovascular functioning, improved glucose control, increased lifespan, reduced muscle loss, reduced hunger, improved metabolism, improved self-image and energy, reduced risk of cancer, and reduced risk of neurodegenerative disease (among others).

12. What are the best foods for me to eat if I am trying to stimulate autophagy?

This is one of the most popular questions that people ask when it comes to autophagy. Many foods stimulate autophagy, but the so-called big four are ginger, green tea, reishi mushrooms, and turmeric/curcumin. These foods are all important in the Ayurvedic Medicine of Asia. Research has shown that their health benefits are so numerous that it is difficult to list them. Many if not most of these benefits can be attributed to their ability to stimulate autophagy in specific cells in the body. These foods generally have anti-cancer benefits, anti-aging benefits, and positive metabolic properties.

13. Is it true that autophagy can help fight cancer?

It has been shown that stimulating autophagy can be effective in treating and preventing several types of cancer, especially colon cancer and lung cancer. This is a general benefit of autophagy stimulation as well as a specific benefit of some stimulators, such as some types of food (see the chapter on foods that stimulate autophagy). Autophagy helps to fight cancer both by triggering cell death in cells before they become cancerous and by helping degrade cancer cells.

14. How should I decide what type of diet I should go on?

Many factors go into the decision of choosing the best diet for you. Many men and women make this decision based on their specific weight loss goals. For example, someone attempting to lose weight quickly might decide to resort to diets that claim to cause dramatic weight loss, like the paleo diet or Atkins diet. In this book, we review diets that trigger autophagy: namely the Ketogenic diet, intermittent fasting, water fasting, and fasting-mimicking diet. The big difference between these diets is how restrictive they are in terms of when you can eat (and to a lesser extent, how much you eat). For most people considering autophagy, the question becomes whether they are healthy enough to withstand a long fast. Some people like to start out with fasting-mimicking diet or water fast rather than jump into a more restrictive type of intermittent fasting diet or Keto.

15. What is fasting-mimicking, and are there any benefits to this type of diet compared to some of the others?

The Fasting Mimicking Diet bears some similarities to other diets in that it closely follows caloric intake and macronutrients. This diet allows dieters interested in reaping the benefits of diets like the Ketogenic diet or intermittent fasting to tap into these without many of the restrictions. The Fasting Mimicking Diet devotes five days out of a 30-day period to caloric restriction similar to what is seen in Keto while the remaining 25 days are less restrictive. The idea here is to trick the body into thinking it is starving. In this situation, the body will mobilize adipose (fat) stores for energy rather than circulating sugar.

16. How often should I fast?

This is a common question for those interested in integrating fasting into their lifestyle and dieting regimens because of the numerous benefits. The answer to this question is that it varies based on age. Some health and fitness gurus argue that it is better for those over the age of 40 to modify traditional intermittent fasting regimens because a slower metabolism with age leads them to benefit more from a modification.

Specifically, those over the age of 40 can benefit from a normal day of eating (i.e. without any intermittent fasting) followed by a longer than normal period of fasting, such as 20 hours. A typical intermittent fasting regimen is 16 hours of fasting and 8 hours of eating in a 24 hour period. In this example, someone over the age of 40 would have a 20 hour period of fasting punctuated by days of normal eating before and after (therefore fasting every other day). This not only allows them to benefit even more greatly from the anti-aging effects of fasting (such as the telomere effect) because of the longer fasting period, but it also allows them to incorporate their altered metabolism into their dieting regimen better. For those under 40, a traditional 16/8 intermittent fasting schedule can work if intermittent fasting is the road you intend to take.

17. Are there any health benefits to fasting for longer periods?

There are. In fact, research has suggested that the greatest impact of autophagy comes when men and women fast for longer periods (at least 18 hours). Indeed, some studies suggest that fasting for even longer periods, as happens in some cultural and religious groups; the anti-aging and anti-cancer effects are even greater. Although greater information is needed for these benefits to be more clearly delineated and understood, some choose to integrate longer periods of fasting one or two times a year into their general regimen of intermittent fasting or water fasting.

18. Can I drink caffeine when I am fasting?

Some recommend avoiding caffeine altogether during a fast. Others argue that caffeine should be avoided because of some of its stimulating effects, but is not prohibited. The general answer is that you can consume this during your fast, although the recommendation is that if you are going to drink caffeine that you should have it earlier in the day. It has been suggested that caffeine throughout the day may be acceptable in younger people, but can cause problems in older individuals. The issues center on catecholamines like adrenaline that is stimulated by caffeine. Stimulating these catecholamines throughout the day can lead to a type of fatigue called adrenal fatigue that can leave you feeling tired and worse for wear. So if you do need your coffee and tea during your days of fasting, make sure you do it earlier in the day.

19. Can I take supplements and vitamins while I am fasting?

The general consensus here is that you should avoid vitamins and supplements altogether during a fast. There are several reasons for this, but a major one is that vitamins and anti-oxidants can screw with your metabolism and therefore undue the autophagy effects of the fast.

20. Are there any recommendations for breaking a fast?

The general recommendation is to focus on foods that are high in protein and fiber. In an abstract sense, this type of diet is what our human bodies expect us to be eating and therefore not only are less of a shock to the system (compared to highly processed foods and grains) but also help us in terms of getting our GI system moving in a positive way. The recommendation for a first meal is 25% of your body weight in grams of protein (so about 42 grams of protein for a 150 lb. individual). Also, a meal high in prebiotic fiber to get the gut flora back to normal is also a good idea. Prebiotic fiber includes things like asparagus, artichoke, and bok choy.

21. Are there any benefits to the Ketogenic diet?

Fasting is regarded as the be-all and end-all when it comes to stimulating autophagy, but dieting and exercise are extremely powerful, and many people live long, healthy lives without having to fast at all (although many people actually "fast" without doing it consciously.

The Ketogenic diet has become very popular very quickly because of the dramatic effects it can have on your body. Many people have gone from obese size to a normal BMI with the Ketogenic diet. The benefits of the Ketogenic diet include a reduction in blood glucose, increase in insulin sensitivity (and reduced insulin levels), improved organ functioning, improved concentration, lower triglyceride levels, lower blood pressure, and lower blood sugar.

22. What are the best ways to induce autophagy?

Autophagy can be induced or stimulated in a variety of ways. Fasting is one of the most reliable ways of stimulating autophagy, and it is recommended by health enthusiasts who have actively studied the best ways to activate this pathway. Fasting can take a variety of forms, including the well-known intermittent fasting, or so-called alternate day fasting, which involves punctuating days of fasting with "normal" days of eating. Dieting and exercise can also be used to predictably stimulate autophagy. The main ways of stimulating this pathway (that will be examined here) include:

- Fasting
- Dieting with the Ketogenic Diet (or similar regimens)
- Exercise, especially HIIT (high-intensity interval training)

23. Are there other types of autophagy that it is useful to know about?

There are several other types of autophagy that have been studied in addition to the main three types. Some of these fall under the three categories of macroautophagy, microautophagy, and chaperone-mediated autophagy, while others can be regarded as standalone pathways. For example, aggrephagy is regarded as a type of macroautophagy. Some lesser-known types of autophagy include.

Zymography: the detection and degradation of granules in the pancreas

Xenography: the degradation of toxic and infectious particles

Ribophagy: the breakdown of ribosomes

Pexography: the breakdown of peroxisomes (a type of organelle)

Aggrephagy: the degradation of cellular protein aggregates in macroautophagy

Conclusion

Autophagy evolved to help you be the streamlined machine that you ought to be. This process aids the body by helping it to degrade components, such as cells, that do not meet the body's high standards and expectations. Autophagy prevents waste by allowing the body to remove components that detract from core functions. Cellular components that are broken down can be reused to build new cells and also can be used for energy.

Indeed, lipolysis in hepatic cells and other areas where adipose tissue is formed represents one of the aspects of autophagy that is of most benefit to those looking to tap into this cellular process. Naturally, this is because many people looking to utilize autophagy are trying to burn fat and lose weight, but it is also because fat breakdown and metabolism represent a major step in the right direction towards improving your health.

In **Autophagy:** *Discover How to Live Healthy and Longer with Your Self-Cleansing Body's Natural Intelligence*, you learned how you can tap into autophagy to achieve a variety of metabolic goals. Autophagy has become quite popular in recent years, but it is easy to get lost in the quagmire of figuring out what precisely it is how to use it. Indeed, as you have seen, autophagy underlies many of the popular diets and therapies that can change your life, including cancer drugs that are being developed as we speak.

In the first chapter, you began your forays into Autophagy and stimulating it by embarking on an in-depth tour of the subject. You learned that this tool to help you live longer and better is happening constantly within your body as part of your body's survival of the fittest order. Autophagy takes place on a cellular level, and it is triggered by several factors that you can learn to stimulate in order to achieve your health and fitness goals. Indeed, many learn that autophagy is crucial to so many processes in the body that their lives improve dramatically merely by tapping into it one form.

There are many benefits to be gained by tapping into autophagy. These benefits extend beyond the realm of weight loss and fitness. Autophagy has been shown incontrovertibly to be influential in immune functioning, cancer-fighting, metabolism, and longevity. Learning what to do with autophagy begins, in part, by learning what it can do for you. Some of the benefits of autophagy include:

- Improved metabolism and insulin sensitivity
- Improved immune functioning
- Improved DNA repair and stabilization
- Anti-aging effects
- Anti-cancer effects
- Improved exercise tolerance

- Improved cardiovascular function
- Improved nervous system functioning
- Protection from neurodegenerative disease
- Protection from infection
- Improved sense of health and wellness
- Improved quality of life

Autophagy is complex, but that should not dissuade you from using this tool to achieve a better, healthier life. Most people want a life free from disease, filled with positive vibes and energy, where they can enjoy the benefits of being slim and feeling healthy. Autophagy can accomplish this for you, and it does in three ways. The three major types of autophagy – macroautophagy, microautophagy, and chaperone-mediated autophagy – were explored, and you were introduced to some subtypes of this process that are also important and which continue to be actively studied.

Naturally, the autophagy discussion would not be complete if the reader did not learn how they can stimulate it in their own body. Autophagy can be triggered in various ways of which the three most important are fasting, dieting, and exercise. These states trigger the body to begin conserving and streamlining processes, which include removing components that are poorly-functioning or dysfunctional. This can include cells that are not up to snuff, but it can also include cancer cells. Autophagy can also be stimulated in other ways, such as by reduced oxygen as happens in exercise.

Dieting is one of the most popular ways to stimulate the process of autophagy in the human body. The dividing line between dieting and fasting is not always clear as most "fasting" that is done to stimulate autophagy includes a diet of one sort or another. In ***Autophagy***: *Discover How to Live Healthy and Longer with Your Self-Cleansing Body's Natural Intelligence,* you learned how water fasting and ketosis diets can be used to stimulate autophagy in powerful ways. Water fasting works because water contains no calories so you are technically fasting while you are drinking it. Ketosis diets like the Ketogenic diet work because they involve placing your body in ketosis, which results in fat stores being mobilized for energy in the form of ketones. This leads to weight loss and other health benefits.

Diets that tap into this metabolic process are perfect for men and women whose goals are focused less on weight loss and more on muscle preservation. Targeted fat loss is just as important to people who are trying to build (and show) their muscle as it is to people who are trying to lose weight. Intermittent fasting is one of the standouts in the world of Autophagy because of its proven success in helping professional athletes, bodybuilders, fitness competitors, and others achieve their personal and professional goals.

Intermittent fasting involves separating periods of eating by fasting. This fasting period can be as long or as short as you want. Some people choose to engage in alternate-day fasting, which involves fasting for 24 hours followed by a day of eating, while others opt for time-restricted feeding in which they break down their day into periods of eating and fasting. The 16/8 protocol, in which 16 hours are spent fasting and eight hours are spent eating in a 24-hour period, is a popular version of this protocol. Intermittent fasting has been attached to a wide variety of health benefits, many of which overlap with the benefits of the process of autophagy as it has been explored in this book.

Foods are a powerful stimulator of metabolic processes in the body. It is not difficult to understand why this is. Your body's basal metabolic rate is altered by your eating behavior. If you eat diets high in carbohydrates, fats, and processed foods, your body's metabolism tends to slow down. If you eat healthier foods that are low in carbs and less processed your metabolic rate rises (which is something that you want). In ***Autophagy:*** *Discover How to Live Healthy and Longer with Your Self-Cleansing Body's Natural Intelligence,* you learned about three superfoods that you can incorporate into your dieting and exercise regimens. Ginger, green tea, turmeric, and reishi mushrooms have been used consumed for centuries because of their positive health benefits, and it turns out that most of these benefits are tied to autophagy.

Mimicking fasting refers to a type of diet that involves stimulating autophagy by tricking the body into thinking that it is fasting. As you learned, fasting is the gold standard for autophagy stimulation. Research suggests that a 7-day fast may be enough to completely clear cancer cells from the body. The fasting-mimicking diet involves consuming low calories over a period of five days. It also is important to keep close track of your macronutrients. This diet is an option for those who have reservations about fasting or are unable to fast.

Some people learn best by absorbing the tricks of the trade-in convenient lists. In chapters nine and ten, you learned the tips that you can use to help you with fasting and to optimize Autophagy. You were familiarized with some of the important terms mentioned in this book to ensure that you were able to get the most out of the information provided here. Autophagy can change your life. All it will take is a little hard work and education on your end. Oh, and a little green tea every now and again doesn't hurt either.

Intermittent Fasting for Women

The A-Z Guide to Weight Loss, Burn Fat and Live Healthier Through the Process of Autophagy. Heal Your Body with an Intermittent, Alternate-Day and Extended Fasting Diet

Written By

Rachel Dash

sources. Please consult a licensed professional before attempting any techniques outlined in this book.

By reading this document, the reader agrees that under no circumstances is the author responsible for any losses, direct or indirect, which are incurred as a result of the use of information contained within this document, including, but not limited to, — errors, omissions, or inaccuracies.

Table Of Contents

Introduction

Congratulations on purchasing *Intermittent Fasting for Women* and thank you for doing so.

Did you know that you can fast your way to a leaner body? Well, fasting is an ancient tradition that has been proven to have many health benefits among them weight loss. This is besides its significance in religious circles and the medical field. Intermittent fasting offers one of the most sought-after solutions to weight and fat loss, especially among women. Additionally, it also has been found to extend life, inhibit insulin resistance, improve the aging process, and reduce inflammation among other benefits.

With the growing popularity of fasting, this book covers intermittent fasting extensively with a particular focus on women. If you have been looking for a lasting weight loss solution, then you need to keep reading to discover the secrets to living a wholesome life by simply changing the way you eat. I explain to you the concept of intermittent fasting and how you can use it as a woman to burn unwanted fat and achieve your personal health goals.

Packed with invaluable information from cover to cover, this book is an ideal wellness tool that will help you turn around your lifestyle. The information contained in this book will no doubt help you to achieve your goals without having to go through a major lifestyle change. By the end of this book, you'll be able to embrace intermittent fasting with confidence and tap into all the benefits it offers. I have no doubt that this book sure will change your life.

Chapter 1: What Is Intermittent Fasting?

For most people, fasting involves going for long periods without food and even drink. This is especially true among those who practice fasting for religious purposes or medical reasons. This is not far from the truth. Fasting involves voluntarily abstaining from any food and drink over a given period. It can either be absolute where you abstain from all liquids and food or both. Intermittent fasting, on the other hand, involves a pattern of eating that alternates between hours of eating and fasting. This means that you get to define your hours of eating and fasting. Ultimately, intermittent fasting is not all about not eating. In fact, the goal is not restricting calories rather, giving your body a break from food to allow for cleansing as opposed to digesting.

The body usually has proteins as well as other structures that either die or become dysfunctional. This is a natural process that is necessary for ensuring optimal health. In fact, when these dead tissues are not eliminated from the body, they result in cell death and contribute to poor cell or organ function. It may become cancerous in extreme cases. Thus, the process of cleansing takes place when the body enters autophagy.

In the medical world, a diagnostic fast may be prescribed to last between 8-72 hours, depending on the age and procedure. This is usually controlled and under the observation of a health caregiver/physician. This fast is useful in facilitating investigations on certain health investigations. In terms of religious fasting, different religions fast for different reasons over different time frames. For instance, Muslims fast in the holy month of Ramadhan during which they fast from dawn to dusk. Christians too fast when they are seeking to have a deeper connection with God.

History of Intermittent Fasting

There are many fad diets that promise to help you lose weight. However, most of these don't produce the results you desire. Over the years, fasting was used as an expression of dissent, therapeutic tool, or a means of attracting a spiritual reward. This was until intermittent fasting began gaining traction among fitness experts for its anti-inflammatory and weight loss benefits. Intermittent fasting promises to be a game-changer as it is backed with scientific evidence. The concept of intermittent fasting was practiced among ancient men who relied on hunting and gathering fruits and wild berries for survival. The lack of advanced storage technology meant that they ate all they gathered and fasted out necessity in moments of scarcity until the time they'd find something to eat. Later on, Greek philosopher Hippocrates, who is also the father of medicine, encouraged fasting for medical reasons. He held that eating when you are sick feeds the sickness. He observed that sick animals fasted, thus speeding up their healing process. It's actually this concept that has been embraced into modern medicine.

On the other hand, intermittent fasting caught the attention of masses after BBC journalist Dr. Michael Mosley fasted every two days a week and shared the results of the transformation he had achieved. This included benefits like rapid weight loss. While you don't necessarily have to count your calories during intermittent fasting, you generally have fewer hours of eating which translates to eating fewer calories. There are several intermittent methods you can follow to achieve the same results depending on your needs. Today, intermittent fasting continues to gain popularity, especially among women who want to lose weight.

What you need to Know Before Jumping into Intermittent Fasting

Although intermittent fasting is fairly safe to practice, there are certain things you need to know before you begin this lifestyle. To begin with, not everyone can practice intermittent fasting, and even for those who can, you need to consult a doctor. You could be having a prevailing health condition that you're not aware of this, and you'll do well to get the green light first. Keep in mind that fasting is not recommended when you're battling a medical condition. Although women too can benefit from intermittent fasting, you need to know that certain groups of women cannot fast while others must approach fasting with caution. You need to get the doctor's nod if you have the following conditions; low blood pressure, diabetes, eating disorders, you're breastfeeding, you're taking medications or are trying to conceive. Ultimately, you must always assess the risks and benefits before making a decision to either embrace intermittent fasting or not.

What to Eat/Drink during Intermittent Fasting

When you're practicing intermittent fasting, you're shifting from your regular 2-3-hour meal times to a shorter defined eating window. While you can eat anything, you need to keep in mind that your body needs nutrients and you must make up for this need during your feasting window. You need to make food choices that will help keep your blood sugar stable. You also must be careful so that you don't end up being nutrient deficient or even being dehydrated. While there isn't a specific dietary recommendation that you should follow during intermittent fasting, it's common for most people to combine it with the ketogenic diet that is low in carbs. If you're wondering about what to eat during your intermittent fasting journey, here are some food suggestions you need to consider when creating your menu, so you don't end up with nutrient shortfalls:

Raspberries

Fiber is an important part of your diet that helps you maintain a regular bowel movement and maintain a feeling of fullness yet it has been found to be a shortfall nutrient by the 2015 – 2020 Dietary Guidelines. An article in nutrients also states that less than 10% of Western populations consume sufficient amounts of whole fruits. Raspberries are high in fiber with a single cup having eight grams of fiber that is able to keep you regular during your fasting window.

Minimally Processed Grains

Carbohydrates are an important part of your nutrition and not an enemy for your weight loss. Since you'll be spending most hours of your day fasting, you must think strategically when it comes to feeding time to get adequate calories without getting too full. While a healthy diet will have a minimal amount of processed foods, you can also include foods like bagels, whole-grain bread, and crackers as they're easily and quickly digested for fast fuel. These are especially great if you train regularly as they give you energy on the go.

Seitan

Incorporating seitan, a plant-based protein that has amazing anti-aging properties into your diet is a perfect way of complementing your intermittent fasting efforts. The EAT-Lancet commission advocates for a reduction in the number of animal proteins you consume. Moreover, one study linked the consumption of red meat to an increase in mortality. Seitan is also known as wheat meat because it can be dipped, baked, and battered in any of your favorite sources.

Wild Caught Salmon

This is one of the most commonly consumed foods across the Blue Zones in five regions in Latin America, Europe, the U.S. and Asia that are popular for lifestyle and dietary choices that are associated with extreme longevity. This fish is high in omega-3 fatty acids DHA and EPA that are brain-boosting.

Potatoes

Just like bread, white potatoes digest fast and with minimal effort from your body. Moreover, when it's paired with a good protein source, it's a perfect post-workout snack that will refuel your muscles. The other benefit that makes potatoes an important staple during intermittent fasting is that once they're cooled, potatoes usually form a resistant starch that is primed to fueling the good bacteria in your gut.

Soybeans

Isoflavones, an active compound in soybeans, has demonstrated to hinder UVB induced cell damage in addition to promoting anti-aging. Thus, you'll do well to include it in your meals during intermittent fasting as it will complement the benefits of autophagy.

Hummus

This is another excellent plant-based protein that is perfect for boosting the nutritional content of staples such as sandwiches. You can be adventurous to make your own but keep in mind the secret to the perfect recipe is tahini and ample garlic.

Vitamin D fortified milk

It's recommended that an average adult takes 1,000 milligrams of calcium daily. This is equivalent to 3 cups of milk per day. Shortening your feeding window significantly reduces the opportunity to take as much milk, therefore, make sure that you also prioritize your consumption of calcium-rich foods. Vitamin D fortified milk is a great choice because it will enhance the consumption of calcium hence help in keeping your bones strong. You can add the milk to cereal, and smoothies drink alongside your meals.

Lentils

These nutrient-packed cereals are high in fiber with about 32% of you total recommended amount of fiber you need per day. In addition, lentils are a good source of iron at about 15% of your daily needs making it especially great among women who are not only active but are also practicing intermittent fasting.

Multivitamins

The mechanism of intermittent fasting for weight loss is based on the time allocated to eating and fasting versus the principle of energy in and energy out. Even then, this conversation seldom highlights the risk of vitamin deficiencies due to the caloric deficit occasioned be fewer feeding hours. As such, you need to make sure that you include plenty of vegetables and fruits to take care of any deficiencies that may arise.

There are numerous other foods that you need to include in your diet during intermittent fasting that include blueberries, olives, nuts, papaya, ghee, avocado, cruciferous vegetables, probiotics, eggs, and whole grains among others. Before you change the way you eat or even alter your diet in a significant way, you need to speak with a health professional just to be sure that it's the best decision based on your health and goals.

What Can I Drink When Fasting?

What can you drink when doing intermittent fasting? Although you must completely abstain from eating food during intermittent fasting, you need to stay hydrated. Here are some of the drinks that you can take during your fasting window:

Water

Proper hydration is one of the important aspects of making sure you maintain a healthy system when fasting. You can drink as much water as possible without breaking your fast. Water is considered to be the best drink during fasting. Water is also full of minerals that are important in restoring the body's mineral and electrolyte balance that occurs during fasting. Abstaining from food for 12-16 hours signals the body to tap into the sugar; glycogen, that is stored in the liver. Consequently, you lose a large volume of electrolytes and fluid as this energy is being burned. Therefore, drinking at least eight glasses of water will promote cognition and blood flow as well as prevent dehydration. It will also promote better muscle and joint support. It can either be carbonated, plain or flavored with a bit of lemon but must not be sweetened. Essentially, you need to drink at least half of your body weight in ounces. This means that if you're weighing 160 pounds, then you should drink at least 80 ounces of water. This is in addition to the other beverages you may be taking. Taking water during intermittent fasting is extremely important because it's a great way of curbing hunger. This makes it much easier to stick to your intermittent fasting protocol without much of a struggle. Taking water also helps in lubricating your joints, regulating your body temperature, and making sure your digestive system stays regular. Water is also instrumental in carrying oxygen as well as nutrients to your cells in addition to flushing out waste from your body and maintaining healthy blood pressure. Drinking water while you're fasting will also increase the production of heat in your body through a process that is known as thermogenesis.

Flavored vs. Carbonated Water. Taking plain water can be a challenge, especially if you're not used to it. Thus, you can consider taking flavored or carbonated water instead. Even then, you must be careful enough to read the labels just to be sure that the water doesn't have sweeteners or sugars as well. This is because taking water containing natural no-calorie sweeteners such as stevia is likely to kick start your sugar carving, thus making it more difficult for you to stick to your fasting plan.

Black Coffee

Taking black coffee during fasting will not break your fast of even get your body out of ketosis. Studies have shown that taking caffeine during fasting can instead increase your metabolism hence promoting weight loss. Black coffee is also handy in curbing appetite; thus; it can help you get through your fast in a more manageable way. Even then, you need to refrain from the temptation of adding cream, syrups and candied flavorings or sugar that are likely to break your fast. Moreover, try not to go overboard with it because taking too much coffee will leave you feeling weak, anxious, and jittery, particularly if you're sensitive to caffeine. Keep in mind that taking coffee late into the night can interfere with the quality of your sleep. When you take coffee on an empty stomach, the caffeine will be assimilated into your bloodstream faster than when you've taken a meal. Therefore, you can stick to taking one or two cups (400mg of caffeine) of black coffee a day.

Tea

Drinking tea during intermittent fasting doesn't break a fast. If anything, tea is a great choice while you're fasting. You may want to try various kinds of tea like green tea which has powerful antioxidants that help in burning calories. Just as with coffee, you can only take tea that has not been sweetened or has cream in it. Although it's not easy to transition to taking unsweetened tea, it gets better with time. In fact, avoiding sugar in your tea can eventually become a lifestyle. If you find it difficult taking unsweetened tea you can begin by reducing the amount of sugar you put in a cup over time until you get to that point where you can do without. The other variation of tea you can also consider is herbal tea.

Apple Cider Vinegar

You can dilute a small amount of apple cider vinegar in water and take without breaking your fast. A 2018 study published in the Journal of Medicinal Food found that apple cider vinegar can promote positive metabolic changes that can help in encouraging weight loss. Consuming apple cider vinegar on a daily basis may also reduce your body's total cholesterol, LDL (bad cholesterol) levels, and triglycerides. Apple cider vinegar also helps in lowering your blood sugar levels while improving digestion. However, this must be diluted in water before taking. Apple cider vinegar contains acetic acid that is potent; hence drinking it without diluting can damage your tooth caramel. It's best to take it before going to sleep.

When doing intermittent fasting, make sure you stay away from sugary drinks, especially during the fasting window. Eating a lot of sugar means that most of it won't be used for energy; rather, it will be broken down and stored as body fat. In addition, introducing sugar into your system will cause your insulin levels and blood sugar to spike, making it difficult to lose weight. What follows the initial spike in blood in your blood sugar is a dramatic drop in energy, prompting you to eat more hence store more fat. For this reason, it's advisable that you avoid sugary drinks like fruit juices, lemonade, soda, and sweetened ice tea even when you're not fasting.

What not to Eat/drink During Intermittent Fasting

Although intermittent fasting emphasizes more on when you eat as opposed to what you eat, it's advisable to stay away from foods that have empty calories when fasting. This is especially true if your goal is to lose weight. These are counterproductive to your weight loss efforts. You can optimize your intermittent fasting for weight loss by being mindful of your food choices. This will help you to stay away from the processed foods that have sugar additives and other undesirable ingredients that improve taste yet have a negative effect on your health. In most cases, sugar may not be included in the ingredients list, but there's a form of substitute that usually has a worse effect than sugar.

Drinks to Avoid During Intermittent Fasting

Diet Soda

One of the frequently asked questions about intermittent fasting is, "can I drink diet soda while intermittent fasting?" Although diet soda doesn't have any carbohydrates, calories or sugar and may seem okay to take when fasting. In fact, it comes across as a perfect alternative to soda, but that's not the case. Diet soda, as well as other diet drinks, are laden with artificial sweeteners that are capable of increasing your craving for sugar and insulin resistance drastically. It also increases your risk of developing diabetes as well as make it hard for you to lose weight. This is backed by a 2015 study that found the fat belly in people who drank diet soda tripled in nine years. Thus, it's best not to take diet drinks at all. However, if you must include them, then make sure you're taking them in moderation.

Juices

Just as with diet soda, there are a lot of misconceptions around the consumption of juices during intermittent fasting. Here's why; fresh juice is a powerhouse of minerals and vitamins. On the other hand, they also contain sugar that is capable of breaking a fast. Well, even though it may come across as a healthy drink option, taking juice during intermittent fasting will no doubt break your fast. This is because in most cases, a glass of juice will have about 100-150 kcal. This means that having a couple of glasses of juice is equivalent to having a meal. Thus, if you must take juice, make sure it's during your eating window.

Alcohol

You should not drink alcohol when fasting. Here is the reason behind it; when you fast, your stomach is left empty because you haven't eaten for a couple of hours. Therefore, when you drink alcohol is absorbed into your bloodstream rapidly. As a result, you are bound to have extreme hangovers, severe dehydration, and increased intoxication. Besides, some alcoholic beverages usually contain calories that will negate the effects of your fast. Adding sweetened beverages only goes to amplify this situation. Thus, you need to avoid alcoholic beverages when fasting altogether.

Intermittent Fasting Compared to Other Diets

We've all tried out a fad diet at some point in life. From a high protein, low carb, keto to extreme calorie restriction to lose weight. Unfortunately, while you initially lose weight, it gradually returns. To achieve long term results, you need to focus on implementing healthy lifestyle choices. This is what makes intermittent fasting unique and more promising than most fad diets. With intermittent fasting, you must learn to make conscious decisions with regard to when you will eat. That is, rather than eliminating certain foods from your diet or even cutting calories; you reduce the window within which you eat. This method of losing weight emphasizes that weight gain/loss is regulated by insulin levels. Thus, rather than restricting calories and even the kind of food you eat, you instead watch the times you eat to create a gap between your eating and fasting windows. The calories you consume will reduce by default because you have a shorter window during which you can eat.

Chapter 2: Understanding Intermittent Fasting for Women

Although both men and women can practice intermittent fasting, women have reported experiencing certain effects relating to hormonal imbalance. Some of the common of these effects include metabolic disturbances, missed period, and in some cases, the early onset of menopause. This chapter explores the effect of intermittent fasting in women and what women can do to make their intermittent fasting experience smooth.

How Intermittent Fasting Affects Women Differently than Men

Despite its benefits, intermittent fasting can result in hormonal imbalances in women when not done properly. This is because, by nature, women are extremely sensitive to the signals of starvation. Thus, when the body senses that it's being starved, then it ramps up the production of hunger hormones ghrelin and leptin. When women experience insatiable hunger, what they're actually experiencing is an increase in the production of these hormones. This is the body's way of protecting a potential fetus even when you're not pregnant.

Calorie restriction may inhibit the production of the female sex hormones resulting in infertility, irregular periods hormonal imbalances, and halt ovulation. As a result, it may affect your menstruation and even cause your ovaries to shrink. In some women, intermittent fasting can also worsen eating disorder like binge eating and anorexia.

This is why it's important for women who are interested in intermittent fasting not to do it for calorie restriction but focus on health and wellness. When you restrict calories for the female body, you may end up with a number of changes like slowed-down metabolism, hormones going out of balance and failure of the body to function at optimum levels. It's also worth noting that intermittent fasting can have different effects on women, depending on their ages. For instance, intermittent fasting isn't a big risk to the overall health of women who are post-menopausal. Even then, pre-menopausal women are likely to experience poor outcomes with moderate or extreme forms of intermittent fasting.

Here's what you can expect when you're fasting:

Emotional instability. This is mostly triggered by the fluctuation of hormones during intermittent fasting. It's particularly common within the first two weeks to about one month into intermittent fasting.

Excessive fatigue. During fasting, you'll experience fatigue as well as muscle weakness because of a decrease in calorie intake. However, this effect is usually elevated in females because of the female body's tendency to rely on glucose for its energy as opposed to the stored fat. The positive side of this is that these effects fade off over time as your body gets accustomed to the changes in your eating pattern.

Hormonal imbalance. This is rather common because transitioning from regular feeding pattern to intermittent fasting can progress into more pressing issues that are linked to genetics. Hormonal imbalances can result in an irregular length of the menstrual cycle, missed periods and blemishes that are difficult to clear.

When done properly, women can experience the many benefits that intermittent fasting offers. Ultimately, you must weigh between the benefits and the risks to determine if it's worthwhile to carry on with intermittent fasting.

How can you Practice Intermittent Fasting Safely

The secret to making intermittent fasting work for you as a woman is by making sure you practice intermittent fasting safely. Keep in mind the following:

Assess your stress levels. Fasting by itself is a form of stress on the body with the potential of causing negative effects. When you start intermittent fasting and notice some signs of hormonal imbalance, you should consider stopping or modifying your fast. By modifying, it can either mean increasing your daily eating window while shortening your fasting window.

Eat fewer calories. If your goal of intermittent fasting is shedding some pounds, you should eat the fewest number of calories you need to maintain your weight during the eating window. This is referred to as maintenance calories. However, if you want to be healthier, make up for the missed meal even if it means going a little over your maintenance calories. Most importantly, take your lifestyle into account before you start a plan.

Start slowly. Regardless of the intermittent plan that you'll opt to start with, make sure you start slowly. When eating, limit your carbs, and push meals to include high amounts of protein and healthy fat.

Generally, women will have more success and less hormonal effect when they follow a shorter fasting window spanning between 12 to 14 hours.

How Women Can Benefit from Intermittent Fasting

Although the most common and sought after intermittent fasting benefit among women is weight and fat loss, there's more. Other benefits of intermittent fasting in women include:

Reproductive health benefits. Studies have linked intermittent fasting to reproductive health benefits in women. A number of health conditions that are related to the endocrine dysfunction in women like Polycystic Ovarian Syndrome (PCOS), metabolic syndrome, and obesity can be improved through intermittent fasting. One study conducted among women with PCOS found that the stress neurohormone levels reduced, thus having a positive effect on physical and mental health. In another study, short-term caloric restriction was found to increase the luteinizing hormone among women with PCOS. This hormone is produced within the pituitary gland and is important in ensuring healthy ovulation patterns. This augurs well with balancing hormones in addition to being a fertility marker.

Metabolic Health. The risk of cardiovascular disease in women increases post-menopause. This is usually because of belly fat, increased LDL cholesterol, and high triglyceride levels. Elevated levels of glucose and insulin are also seen as factors. Studies have found that intermittent fasting can have a significant improvement in metabolic health in women with these symptoms, thus eliminating the risk of cardiovascular diseases.

Musculoskeletal health benefits. Chronic pain disorders have become common among women in their 40's. These include arthritis, osteoporosis, chronic back pain, fibromyalgia, and more. Intermittent fasting has been found to be effective when it comes to supporting musculoskeletal conditions among women.

One study found that intermittent fasting affects the parathyroid hormone that is critical to improving bone health and is also helpful in cases of rheumatoid arthritis (RA). Fasting improves the symptoms of intestinal permeability, thus decreasing food intolerance. This, in turn, results in a decrease in inflammatory markers and prevention of the vicious circle of inflammation that rheumatoid arthritis is part of. Weight loss also supports musculoskeletal health because fasting promotes normalization of hormones that determine your weight; fasting can be a great remedy to musculoskeletal health because of weight loss.

Mental Health. According to the World Health Organization (WHO), women have higher rates of mental health disorders, especially anxiety and depression. One of the reasons behind this has a lot to do with stressors with the most common one being food. Weight and our outer appearance have been packaged as something we need to fix constantly. Unfortunately, this also affects how we feel about ourselves, leaving us with so many insecurities. Intermittent fasting helps harness inherent health as well as simplify the mental burden of wondering what to eat. Fasting also helps to deal with the hormonal instability in menopause that is also linked to tension, emotional pressure, anxiety, and depression. Overall, fasting helps to improve your mental status and self-esteem, reduce depression and anxiety while promoting social functioning.

Other pros of intermittent fasting include an increase in lean muscle mass, sustainable weight loss, more energy, an increase in cell stress response, a reduction in inflammation and oxidative stress, improved insulin sensitivity and an increase in the production of neurotrophic growth factor. Intermittent fasting is an exciting way of making lifestyle changes to your pattern of eating and taking charge of your health while at it. This is particularly great for women who have struggled with weight and its related health issues for years.

Cons of Intermittent Fasting

Some of the cons that are linked to intermittent fasting include the following:

- Fertility issues
- Difficulty sleeping
- Shrinking of the ovaries
- Metabolic stress
- Anxiety
- Irregular periods

Due to the interconnected nature of hormones, when one hormone is thrown off balance, it affects the others negatively. If you're wondering if it's still worth practicing intermittent fasting the other is yes. You only need to figure out the right approach. Remember, intermittent fasting is meant to complement a healthy lifestyle and diet.

Intermittent Fasting Post Menopause

Getting into menopause is not usually an exciting time because of the many symptoms that you're likely to experience. This can be anything from weight gain, elevated temperature, low self-esteem, interrupted sleep, cravings, mood swings, and hot flashes, among others. Dealing with some or all these symptoms can be overwhelming, making your transition difficult. Studies have shown that intermittent fasting is giving menopausal and post-menopausal women great results. Post-menopausal women have been found to lose twice as much weight as premenopausal women because of better adherence to diets. These findings show that intermittent fasting is particularly beneficial for women post-menopause.

More specifically, intermittent fasting is a great way of reducing belly fat and preventing weight gain not only during but also after menopause. Fasting intermittently can also help in lowering the risk of diabetes by decreasing blood pressure, blood cholesterol, as well as enhancing insulin resistance.

It's important to keep in mind that not every intermittent fasting method is suitable for you. During menopause, your body is usually more sensitive to any changes that may come. So, it's advisable that you build upon the length of your fasting window gradually. Therefore, make sure you identify the method that works best for you. Test out to see if fasting and taking only fluids will ease or increase your menopause symptoms. If the symptoms increase, then it's best to stop immediately, take a break before trying another method. Here's how to get started:

- Start with 12-hour eating and 12-hour fasting window
- Increase your fasting window gradually to 16 hours
- Avoid an extreme fasting window of more than 16 hours
- Make sure you stay hydrated by taking lots of fluids during your fasting window
- Build up with gentle exercise while paying attention to how your body feels
- Get some fresh air

Some women have found drinking alcohol and eating sugary foods later at night are more likely to induce night sweats and hot flushes. For others, eating clean and early causes menopause symptoms to disappear. The benefits of intermittent fasting may have an impact on your menopause symptoms. Nonetheless, everyone is different; therefore, it's important to listen to your body. If you can't sleep and are feeling anxious, then stop fasting. Remember, intermittent fasting is just one of the many healthy lifestyle options that can help you in menopause. Focus on eating unprocessed foods, drinking lots of water, and staying active.

Intermittent Fasting in Pregnant Women

If you're using intermittent fasting to increase fertility and you become pregnant, make sure you work closely with your medical practitioner to make adjustments to your eating schedule. This is important because you need to nurture your body through a healthy and safe pregnancy. Although intermittent fasting isn't appropriate in pregnancy, there are variations as well as companion eating styles to intermittent fasting that are. For instance, it's not just safe to restrict refined and processed grains while increasing healthy fats, it's strongly suggested. In fact, most of the leading dieticians inclined towards pregnancy and fertility recommend a carefully designed very low carbohydrate and high-fat diet for expectant women who have gestational diabetes.

Can Intermittent Fasting Extend Fertility in Women?

Studies done in mice and worms suggest that intermittent fasting can contribute towards extending fertility in women. This conclusion is based on the premise that restricting food helps to improve the egg quantity and quality that are linked to aging. The first study which was performed in adult female mice found that the egg produced by these mice upon calorie restriction were more likely to develop into embryos when fertilized. Another study performed in worms found that the worms had inactive NHR-49 gene reproductive recovery and fertility post starvation. This process is believed to be the same in humans, even though it hasn't been tasted. It's still not clear how much caloric restriction is required to activate this system in human beings. However, if the underlying signaling molecules can be identified along with ways of manipulating them, then it could help in treating fertility problems and extend the of female reproductive lifespan. Studies also reveal that as little as 5-10% weight loss usually has significant clinical benefits in improving psychological outcomes, metabolic features (risk factors for cardiovascular diseases and insulin resistance), and reproductive features (ovulation, fertility, and menstrual cyclicity)

Intermittent Fasting Risks for Women

Before getting into intermittent fasting, you need to know that this healthy practice isn't risk-free. You need to have a discussion with your physician to determine the health risks that fasting could have on you. Some existing medical conditions, your age, or even medication you may be taking can be risk factors. In most cases, dosing is closely scheduled around your regular meal times. Moreover, it's advisable that you avoid fasting altogether if you're breastfeeding or you're underweight. Women who are developing an eating disorder must also refrain from fasting because it can only get worse.

Most women agree to have experienced the same negative effects of intermittent fasting as men. These effects range from muscle weakness, dehydration, initial loss of muscle tone, and headaches. Additionally, women with a history of irregular periods have experienced symptoms of infertility after fasting for a considerable period. This is especially common in women who lose fat dramatically in the initial weeks of intermittent fasting. However, most of these changes aren't permanent. Most women tend to have their fertility restored soon after they stop fasting. Medical experts advise women who are hoping to get pregnant to avoid fasting.

Should Women Practice Intermittent Fasting?

Fasting is a great option to pursue if you want to lose weight or lead a healthy life altogether. Although most women tolerate fasting, others have to deal with hormonal imbalance when they do intermittent fasting. Fasting may also result in the loss of periods or even interfere with the production of the thyroid hormone posing a great risk, especially if you have autoimmune issues. If you happen to experience any of these issues, you can consider opting for the gentler intermittent fasting methods. You can choose to fast for non-consecutive days or lesser duration of between 12 and 14 hours. You'll still enjoy the benefits of intermittent fasting even though your hormones may still be affected. If you feel good doing the shorter fasts several times a week, you can increase the length of your fast with time. Intermittent fasting could amazingly well for some people and worse for others. Therefore, you need to listen to your body. At the end of the day, your physical, emotional, and mental well-being is most important.

Chapter 3: What Makes Intermittent Fasting the Best Way to Lose Weight

This is the question most people ask before jumping into the intermittent fasting bandwagon. The reason is simple. There has been a lot of buzz around intermittent fasting that it can become difficult to tell it apart from other weight loss diet fads. Intermittent fasting isn't a product; rather, it involves a lifestyle change that requires you to review the times you eat so that you're alternating between periods of fasting and eating. Generally, you'll have more hours of fasting compared to your hours of eating. As a result, you'll experience fat loss because your body is burning and using the stored fat for its fuel when you're in the fasted state. You don't have to make any drastic changes to your lifestyle like the foods you eat or even take chemicals or supplements to speed up the manifestation of the benefits.

Unlike many diet fads you may have tried before, intermittent fasting continues to deliver results for many people. The secret to succeeding with this method of health and wellness is to begin gradually, listen to your body, and make adjustments where necessary. Interestingly, intermittent fasting isn't based on restricting calories. It also doesn't dictate the kind of food you should eat. Instead, you eat your foods normally, so you don't have to give up some foods. Calorie restriction takes place naturally since you have a shorter feeding window. This pattern of feeding helps you to live a healthy lifestyle. This is unlike most diets that leave you with the temptation to eat more than you did before hence resulting in weight gain. Intermittent fasting is easy to follow through because all you need to do is pay attention to when you eat. Moreover, you're free to take fluids during your fasting window, so that eliminate the possibility of binge eating during the feasting window. There are various disadvantages of eating continually, particularly those foods containing free radicals. Thus, taking a rest from eating allows your body to rest from digestive processes. If you're not sure about embracing intermittent fasting for weight loss, here are some reasons you should consider this pattern of eating over dieting:

It's convenient. Diets can be demanding. In fact, one of the main reasons why most people abandon diets is because of the inability to follow through. Meeting various life's daily demands that require your attention alongside dieting can be a huge challenge. Intermittent fasting frees up the time you'd have spent preparing meals because you're essentially skipping a number of meals in a day. This means you have fewer instances of decision making. Moreover, you don't have to worry about moving away from your usual food choices as long as you're emphasizing on eating healthy whole foods. This is contrary to most diets that happen to be complex and expensive altogether, yet they don't produce the desired results.

Fasting strengthens your will power. Your intermittent fasting success is dependent on self-discipline. Intermittent fasting calls for you to be able to resist food even when you're tempted to eat. In the long run, this strengthens your capacity to stay focused and ignore distractions not just with food but other areas of your life as well. This eventually improves your ability to stay focused and focus on achieving your goals. When you fast, you become more alert and focused; thus, you can ignore any distractions that may come your way to achieve a set goal.

It's a great way to transition into a healthy lifestyle. Let's face it, most people find it difficult to stick to eating unprocessed foods even though they desire to. After all, processed foods are easily accessible, and they taste better. Intermittent fasting is a great way towards a lifestyle change because while it doesn't explicitly spell out the foods you should eat or avoid, you'll have better results when you include healthy foods in your meals. When your body adjusts to a shorter feeding window, you eliminate the temptation of eating junk food when hunger strikes.

It saves you money and time. Diets are generally expensive because you have to shop for specific food items and follow the menu to the latter in order to get certain results. This is in addition to the time you'll spend in meal preparation throughout the day. This is usually draining and a burden to your lifestyle. By fasting, you get to save resources and time.

A structured way of eating. When you're on a normal eating regimen, you're likely to keep on snacking mindlessly. In fact, you'll be surprised to learn that there's always something you can nibble on. Eventually, you end up putting on weight. Fasting helps you to have a structured pattern of eating.

Bigger meals are more satiating. Unlike the regular eating regimen where you're constantly thinking about food, intermittent fasting lets you have bigger meals which are more satiating because you'll be fuller for longer.

You can incorporate it into your social gatherings. When you're on a diet, it's unlikely that you'll be able to fit into social gatherings without having to worry about what you'll eat. With intermittent fasting, you can work out your schedule in a way that your feeding window falls within the time when you're most likely to attend social gathers. This way, you won't have to miss out on special occasions or even go out with friends.

You can fast and travel the world. If you love to globe-trot, you don't have to worry about putting off your intermittent fasting plan. Actually, intermittent fasting offers you a lot of flexibility that allows you to fast wherever you are. This means that you can maintain your lifestyle while at the same time, be able to enjoy new experiences and cuisines. Most importantly, you don't have to give up on this new way of life because you're traveling.

Heightened hunger awareness. Feelings of thirst and hunger are processed by the same part of your brain. As such, it's common to find that you're eating after every two hours because of other reasons that are manifesting as hunger. This could be feelings of boredom, stress, sadness, or happiness. Did you know that the smell of food can make you assume you're hungry? When you fast, your hunger awareness is heightened so that you actually know what it feels like to be hungry and can differentiate between the feel of hunger that is linked to other factors.

Improved quality of sleep. Most people who adopt the intermittent fasting lifestyle are motivated by the desire to shed excess weight. This might also be a case for you. What you don't know is that with it comes other benefits like better sleep. The reason for this is simple. When you're fasting, your body will mostly digest food before you go to bed. When your fat and insulin levels are kept in check, the quality of your sleep improves.

What Intermittent Fasting Does to your Body

Imagine having to wait for 16-18 hours before having your next meal. Well, that pretty much puts intermittent fasting into perspective - time-restricted eating. Understanding the science behind intermittent fasting is the first step towards reaping the benefits it promises. When you eat, your body releases insulin that is instrumental in the conversion of sugars into energy. The glucose that is not used is stored as fat. When you fast, you're naturally restricting calories; therefore, insulin is not released. What this means is that you can't lose weight unless your insulin levels go down. This explains why eating small meals all through the day isn't helpful when it comes to weight loss. When your insulin levels go down, it causes your body to respond by tapping into the fat stores in the liver and muscles for energy. When it exhausts these sources, it enters a state known as ketosis. This is where the liver breaks down fat to produce ketones that are used as a source of energy. Moreover, ketones are also known for their role in lowering appetite, reducing oxidative stress and inflammation levels. Ketones are also a source of a number of other benefits like a reduction in the risk factors for conditions like type 2 diabetes and heart disease.

Benefits of Intermittent Fasting

Intermittent fasting continues to take the health and fitness world by storm ostensibly because of its benefits. Most people who have tried losing weight over the years are often drawn to intermittent fasting because of the benefits it offers then go beyond losing weight. These benefits include the following:

Accelerated weight and fat loss. A 2017 study that was published in the journal of research found that intermittent fasting will help you lose weight even without having to count calories. This is based on the fact that during intermittent fasting, you have a shorter window within which you can eat your meals and achieve your daily calorie consumption. Eventually, this will reduce your calorie consumption naturally because it's utterly impossible to squeeze 4000 calories in your meals within a 4-hour window. This means that you will have a calorie deficit leading to significant loss of weight. In scientific terms, when you reduce your consumption of food, your blood insulin decreases paving the way for the process of breaking down fat for glucose to give energy. Eventually, your levels of cholesterol and triglycerides decreases. Even then, you must recognize that intermittent fasting is not a magic bullet for obesity and weight loss. Rather, it's a realistic approach that you can consider.

Improved cardiovascular health. Heart disease is a leading killer disease in the world. A study investigating the health benefits of intermittent fasting among non-obese individuals found a significant reduction in the level of triglyceride in men. On the other hand, women experienced an increase in good

HDL cholesterol. This change was attributed to a 4% decline in body fat. Intermittent fasting ameliorates risk factors linked to a number of heart diseases by inducing stress resistance that has a cardioprotective effect.

Increased longevity. It may sound ironical that abstaining from food can actually increase longevity. Fasting has proven to increases the lifespan of various organisms like yeast and worms, among others. While intermittent fasting doesn't explicitly focus on calorie reduction, it shortens the feeding window, which eventually has an effect on the number of calories you can consume in a day. As a result, you get to enjoy better insulin sensitivity and a decline in the free radical damage to proteins and DNA, the body's cellular components. The result of this is lowered heart rate and blood pressure as well as a decline in incidences of spontaneous and induced tumors. Your body also becomes more resistant to neurodegenerative diseases. When you're in the fasted state, your body responds by producing various chemicals as a protective measure. These chemicals shield you from the side effects of fasting in addition to helping you fight depression and anxiety. They also help the body to become resistant to stress, thus slowing down the aging process; thus, promoting longevity.

Improved brainpower. Intermittent fasting boosts neuronal usefulness that frequently diminishes with the progression of age. As you advance in age, your dendritic spines begin diminishing. This influences the productivity of neural procedures significantly. Intermittent fasting will counteract the decrease of the dendritic spines density. A study of rats that were on an ordinary eating regimen revealed a 38% decrease in the number of dendritic spines. On the other hand, the rats that were on intermittent fasting had a close insignificant distinction in a youthful rodent that following 24 hours. It's worth noting that the rats also had improved learning capacities. The decrease in calorie consumption that is activated by intermittent fasting expands the procedure of neurogenesis, which is basically the arrangement of new brain cells, while likewise shielding the neurons from death. Moreover, it invigorates the generation of Brain-Derived Neurotropic Factor (BDNF), a protein that is connected to the expansion during neurogenesis. This hinders the neuron degenerations and aging. The impact on neurogenesis supports functional recuperation just as the mending of any harm to the spinal cord, notwithstanding whether intermittent fasting is introduced before or after injury.

Increased fitness training. Fasting can complement your training efforts in a number of ways. The most common ones are hormone production, muscle development, and their connection to fasting. Neurotransmitters play an important role in connecting the body, brain, and senses to provide immediate responses. On the other hand, hormones connect the messages that are gathered in the body with sustained long-term directives. The directives only slow down when the production of the hormone slows down. The growth hormone usually slows when we're past the adolescent growth phase. This is a problem among middle-aged adults who are discovering the importance of leading a healthy lifestyle and are into working to bulk, train, or tone their bodies. To understand the theory of intermittent fasting, think about a time when the hunting season is approaching, and you're running out of food, you'll need stronger muscles and a lean body. This explains why more of the growth hormone is produced during intermittent fasting. This enhanced growth response was revealed in a 2011 study where hormones, along with inflammatory responses, came together, increasing the rate of wound healing in mice subjected to intermittent fasting.

Decreased persistent illnesses. Obesity and painful arthritic conditions are inflammatory diseases that are common today. Intermittent fasting reduces unnecessary inflammation and the risk of developing diseases associated with it. This means that intermittent fasting is able to improve long term health. A number of intermittent fasting methods have been tested to determine their effectiveness in disease control, and the results have been the same. A 2013 analysis of studies and instances where individuals followed guided fasting the restricted eating at certain times and the conclusion was that fasting is linked to prevention or deceleration of most chronic inflammatory diseases. A further review found that fasting can modulate risk factors effectively, thus preventing the onset of diseases.

Better immune and inflammatory responses. The immune system is complex, yet it's what keeps the body from yielding to the onslaught of pathogens around you daily. However, it also could turn against the body and launch an attack at any time. Inflammation refers to the gathering of the white blood cells as well as other immune responses to eliminate and attack any threats to the body. A 2012 study on 50 people who observed Ramadhan, to analyze how their bodies responded to fasting, revealed that there was less inflammation during fasting. This study also noted diastolic and systolic blood pressure, the percentage of body fat and body weight reduced significantly. This decline was only notable when the participants fasted as the markers were higher again when they ceased fasting.

Reduced risk of cancer. Cancer is a dreadful disease that is characterized by the uncontrolled growth of cells. Intermittent fasting is a great step towards slowing down the progression and development of cancer cells. When done alongside chemotherapy, intermittent fasting can slow the progression of skin cancer and breast cancer by increasing the levels of tumor-infiltrating lymphocytes; the cells that are sent by the immune system to attack the tumor.

Intermittent fasting does a lot for your body. Some are obvious, while others are more surprising. This is because by switching to intermittent fasting, you're upgrading your performance in a number of ways.

Chapter 4: Intermittent Fasting and Aging

The search for eternal youth has been in the human imagination since ancient Greece times. A peek at Greek mythology found that youth was more prized compared to immortality. Thus, it's not surprising that high profile celebrities and countless entrepreneurs are embracing intermittent fasting to combat the effects of aging. Apart from weight and fat loss, intermittent fasting continues to gain traction because of its anti-aging benefits. Interestingly, not so many people understand the connection between fasting and its anti-aging effects.

Before we look at the relationship between fasting and aging, it's important to understand the concept of multi-day and micro fasting. Short term fasting protocols where calories are not consumed for at least 16 hours offer many independent benefits. These micro-fasts support metabolic health by lowering insulin levels, improving glycemic control, and controlling body weight. Other fasting benefits include increased brain-derived neurotrophic factor (BDNF) signaling in the brain, cardiovascular support, and lower risk of cancer recurrence. On the other hand, prolonged fasts of more than 48 hours stimulate different physiological changes that present unique fasting benefits relating to functional areas that include healthy aging, longevity, and immune strength.

The Anti-Aging Benefits of Calorie Restriction

Calorie restriction is one of the most efficient interventions for combating aging. Traditional calorie restriction usually reduces calories by between 20 and 40% that is not recommended for performance and is not popular among biohackers because of the mental distraction that comes with it.

Research on calorie restriction in both animals and humans has clarified the mechanisms of aging that were unknown. According to a paper published in clinical interventions of aging, calorie restriction supports the five main mechanisms underlying the process of healthy aging. These are:

- Cell proliferation: IGF and TOR (Specifically mTOR)
- Inflammation: NF-kB
- Mitochondrial physiology: AMPK/SIRT
- Autophagy: FoxO
- Antioxidants: Nrf2

It's important to note that these mechanisms are interrelated. Humans and aging are complex systems

Cell proliferation: IGF-1 and TOR (mTOR). Cell proliferation is used in this context in reference to the tendency of human the human system to be in an anabolic state with the presence of calories. The presence of caloric abundance that is a common feature in industrialized countries means that cells are constantly in an anabolic state. Caloric restriction is able to cause a shift in the balance within the system through stimulation of catabolic pathways. The two pathways that are crucial in this process are the mammalian target of rapamycin (mTOR) and insulin-like growth factor 1 (IGF-1). Both mTOR and IGF-1 are nutrient sensors that regulate cellular resources based on the availability of calories. When you fast, a reduction in the number of calories leads to the downregulation of both mTOR and IGF-1 signaling for the organelles and cells to be repurposed and recycled.

According to the paper on Clinical Interventions in Aging, a reduction in mTOR signaling has been confirmed to extend the lifespan of different organisms. Thus, mTOR inhibition has been identified as a mechanism that guarantees longevity while the availability of rapamycin, along with other mTOR inhibitors makes the pathway a valuable target for interventions that extend healthspan. Since mTOR is a protein sensor hence eating fat only can positively modulate mTOR.

Inflammation: NF-kB. Inflammation is the body's biological mechanism that occurs naturally when your immune system detects a threat like such as a toxic compound, damaged molecule, or even pathogen. However, if inflammation occurs too often or even gets out of control, it can lead to chronic inflammation in the body that contributes to tissue damage or even disease.

As the human body ages, there tends to be cumulative damage throughout the body. Immune receptors recognize this damage by stimulating the productions of numerous proinflammatory molecules. In cases where the damage is so great, the inflammation becomes chronic accompanying a number of age-related diseases or may be contributing to them. Interestingly, inflammation by itself is not bad. If anything, acute inflammation is usually part of healing. However, there's evidence suggesting that chronic inflammation that is commonly referred to as age-related inflammation can be associated with poor health biomarkers. Calorie restriction usually inhibits nuclear factor kB (NF-kB) that exerts the anti-inflammatory effect. *NF-kB* is believed to be the main regulator of inflammation. Therefore, by reducing its activity, you are simply downregulating most parts of the proinflammatory signaling.

According to animal models, the anti-inflammatory effect is capable of producing cognitive enhancing capabilities. One study considered fasting to be a form of eustress, a beneficial form of stress versus distress, which refers to the negative stressors of life that accelerate the aging process. This study came to the conclusion that intermittent fasting caused a notable decrease in the plasma inflammatory factors. Thus, intermittent fasting could improve your cognitive function as well as preserve the brain from distress through regulation of inflammatory response pathway. Engaging in multi-day fasting will help in achieving incredible levels of both physiological and psychological stress.

Mitochondrial physiology: AMPK/SIRT. Mitochondria refer to the organelles that are found in a cell. They have an important role in the production of ATP (cellular energy) letting the cells to do more work. This work can be physical labor, as in the case of muscle cells. It could also be in terms of cognitive tasks as in the increase with brain cells. Aging hampers the general quality of the mitochondrial network through the reduction of the dysfunctional/ damaged mitochondria and subsequent generation of new mitochondria in what is referred to as mitochondrial biogenesis. Calorie restriction supports these processes with the result being a higher quality of the mitochondrial network.

There are two pathways that are usually linked to mitochondrial support are sirtuins (SIRT genes) and AMP-dependent kinase (AMPK). These pathways are quite sensitive to shifts in NAD+ and NADH ratio. Calorie restriction increases the rate of NAD+ accumulation which in effect activate sirtuins and AMPK. The fact that sirtuins need NAD to perform their enzymatic activity connects metabolism to aging-related diseases and aging.

The value of NAD+ / NADH to the sirtuins and AMPK pathways is the reason why the popularity of oral supplementation of precursors has grown. Both sirtuins and AMPK are critical to mitochondrial biogenesis as well as the process of mitophagy, which involves mitochondrial recycling and removal of the dysfunctional organelles that come with aging. Thus, they help in maintaining a mitochondrial network that is younger.

When the cells are deprived of glucose as they normally would in the case of extended fasting, or after intense exercise, the production of ATP drops initially. When AMPK senses a decrease in ATP, it reduces utilization of energy while upregulating many processes that take place to replenish ATP. As a result, the mitochondria and cell are better able to make ATP in the future. The AMPK pathway is activated by calorie restriction in many tissues in animal models. However, the involvement of this mechanism in humans during caloric restriction is not studied. Sirtuins also play an important role in aging as a biological stress sensor. An increase in the expression sirtuins in yeast promotes longevity.

Autophagy: FoxO. During autophagy, a number of cleansing mechanisms take place to remove the old cell membranes, cellular junk, and organelles that have accumulated over time and are likely to hinder optimal mitochondrial and cellular performance. As the old and broken parts of the cells are being removed, the growth hormone that is amplified during fasting signals the body to begin producing new replacements. The result of this process is renovating and recycling of the cells. mTOR induces the activation of forkhead box (FoxO) proteins. Mitophagy and autophagy are FoxO-dependent. This suggests this transcriptional molecule is an integral aspect of these processes.

Antioxidants: Nrf2. As you age, there is an increase in the reactive oxygen species (ROS) while the natural antioxidant defenses decrease. Over time, this imbalance becomes greater; thus, the damage accumulates while the mitochondrial dysfunction becomes prevalent. The normal production of oxidants in particular cell types is important in the regulation of pathways (ROS are important in some signaling processes); hence, it's important to find the right balance. The right balance might be crucial in the optimization of mitochondrial performance in what is referred to as mitohormesis. The idea behind this that the body only needs just the right amount of ROS because too little will result in a performance that is subpar while high amounts will cause damage. This is important for those tissues that rely on the production of large amounts of ATP for metabolism that includes brain, heart, and muscle.

The understanding from mitohormesis is that there's a need for a certain amount of ROS to trigger adaptive responses that upregulate your antioxidant defenses. Calorie restriction activates nuclear factor (erythroid-derived 2) such as Nrf2 that is a regulator of cellular resistance to oxidants. This protein promotes antioxidant defenses through the following:

- Regeneration of the oxidized proteins and cofactors that are mainly re-growing more of the good old stuff.
- Catabolism of peroxides and superoxide, getting rid of the bad stuff.
- Increase in redox transport (Increase inefficiency of existing machinery).
- Synthesis of the reducing factors creating new good stuff.

Even then, Nrf2 is not the only mechanism that promotes antioxidant support ant defenses. All five mechanisms are interrelated; hence, they support each other across the human system that is complex.

Fasting for Lifespan and Healthspan

Lifespan refers to the duration of time we live. On the other hand, healthspan is the length of time you're functional and healthy and not just alive. Calorie restriction influences and is valuable for both healthspan and lifespan. Unfortunately, it's common to focus on lifespan at the detriment of the quality of your life within longevity and aging space. On the contrary, the length of time you're functional and healthy is linked to a higher quality of life. Healthspan can be mediated by various factors that include dietary interventions and social interactions. It's more valuable to emphasize healthspan than lifespan.

Damage Accumulation vs. Programmed

There's a debate between the importance of damage accumulations and programmed aging. Even then, it's important to recognize the complexity of the human system in understanding physiological debates. Programmed aging is all about the changes in the manner in which genes are expressed in aging. Some of these changes are overexpressed, while others are under-expressed. Damage accumulation is characterized by mitochondrial and cellular damage over time. Both damage accumulation and programmed aging occur at the cellular level with each amplifying the effects of the other. That is, how the changes in gene expression accelerate damage accumulation and on the other hand, how damage accumulation affects a cell's ability to have healthy gene expression.

Anti-aging Benefits of Intermittent Fasting

The scientific overview of mechanisms involved with longevity and aging is important beyond the context of fasting. These mechanisms inform nootropics as well as other techniques that can support healthy aging. While we have taken a peek at most of the benefits of intermittent fasting, it's important to note that there are more ways through which you can trigger some of the responses. Some of the benefits occur during the fasting period, but others occur when you start eating. Here are three ways intermittent fasting helps you to live longer:

Hormesis

Evidence has proven that regular intermittent fasting will help cells to become more resilient to any form of cellular stress. Cellular resilience is caused by the hormesis process, which simply describes the biological responses to stress. Intermittent fasting is a form of hormesis; hence, too much fasting would lead to catabolization of muscle tissue and eventually death. However, a little stress from fasting on a daily basis can help to avoid negative effects and instead produce positive biological responses that increase resilience to oxidative stress.

Intermittent fasting increases ketones

When your body is in the fasted state, it's deprived of glucose that comes from the consumption of protein and carbohydrates. The body prefers to draw energy from glucose, but this changes when you fast. In the absence of glucose, the body breaks down fat stored in the liver that it then turns into ketones which is an available source of energy. Ketones are shuttled to the mitochondria where they're used as fuel for muscles, heart, and brain. Even then, certain parts of your body cannot utilize ketones and only require glucose. This glucose is supplied by breaking down protein and fat glycerol through gluconeogenesis. Ketones have some anti-aging benefits. Take the example of Alzheimer's disease.

Fasting triggers autophagy

The process of autophagy will slow down the ability to recycle cells that are under stress. Fasting activates and increases autophagy that in turn, slows down the rate of aging as the body is primed to combat stress. When you're fasting, and your insulin levels drop effectively increasing autophagy.

Overall, intermittent fasting is a simple intervention that has profound benefits that go beyond weight loss. When you eat within a defined window every day, you activate a number of anti-aging pathways. Ultimately, you also must take into account other factors like healthy eating and proper hydration.

Chapter 5: Intermittent Fasting and Autophagy

Efforts to lose weight have shifted from dieting to fasting. Voluntarily going for extended periods without meals is a perfect way to shed bodyweight. The success of intermittent fasting to weight loss is linked to autophagy.

What is autophagy?

Autophagy refers to the body's way of eliminating cells that are damaged to allow for the regeneration of newer cells that are healthier. The word is derived from two words 'auto' meaning self and 'phagy' meaning to eat. Thus, autophagy means self-eating. This process is a great self-preservation mechanism that allows the body to get rid of the dysfunctional cells while recycling some parts of these cells to facilitate a process of cellular repair and cleaning. The term autophagy was coined by Christian de Duve, a Nobel Prize-winning scientist. This process was first described by researchers in 1962 after observing an increase in the number of lysosomes in rat liver cells after infusing glucagon.

The main role of autophagy is removing debris and self-regulating to ensure optimal smooth function. That is, it recycles and cleans simultaneously. This process also promotes adaptation and survival as a response to toxins and stressors that tend to accumulate within the cells. Over time, the cells in your body become old and junky necessitating a replacement or removal. During autophagy, other than killing the cell, some parts of the cell can be replaced. That is, sub-cellular organelles, along with other cellular debris, are removed. This process takes place when the old cells are sent to the lysosome that is a specialized organelle with enzymes that degrade the proteins. During autophagy, the damaged subcellular parts and the unused proteins are marked for destruction before being sent to the lysosomes where the process is finalized.

Types of Autophagy

There are three different kinds of autophagy that include microautophagy, macroautophagy, and chaperone-mediated autophagy. Macroautophagy is the most common type that is an evolutionarily conserved catabolic process that involves the formation of vesicles (autophagosome) which engulf the cellular organelles and macromolecules.

Microautophagy.

Microautophagy refers to the process of sequestration of the cytosolic components directly by the lysosomes through invaginations within their membrane. During microautophagy, fragments and macromolecules of the cell membranes are captured by the lysosome. This paves the way for the digestion of proteins by the cells whenever there's a shortage of building material or energy. Microautophagy processes are non-selective and would normally take place under normal conditions. In some cases, organoids may be digested during this process.

Macroautophagy.

This is the most common type of autophagy. The macroautophagy process involves the degradation of cellular contents by lysosomes before being recycled. The autophagosomes, which are double-membrane structures then enclose the cellular material after which they fuse them with the lysosomes.

Chaperone mediated autophagy

This process involves the selection of soluble cytosolic proteins in a process that is chaperone dependent. These proteins are targeted to lysosomes after which they are translocated directly across the lysosome membrane for degradation.

What Activates Autophagy?

Although drug companies are working towards creating a medical solution that can stimulate autophagy, intermittent fasting is the only proven way to stimulate autophagy. Two main pathways are involved when the body is nutrient deficient;

AMPK or AMP-activated protein kinase that useful in maintaining energy homeostasis and activating the backup fuel mechanisms of your body.

mTOR that is crucial in the regulations of nutrients that affect cellular growth, anabolism, and protein synthesis. When mTOR is activated, the process of autophagy is suppressed; on the contrary, when it is dormant, it promotes autophagy.

Both AMPK and mTOR are in harmony with the presence of nutrients in your body. These two pathways help the body to determine if they will activate a growth response or go into autophagy.

Generally, the main autophagy activator is nutrient deprivation. Glucagon is the opposite of insulin. Thus, when glucagon goes down, the insulin goes up. When you go without food for a lengthy period, your glucagon levels go up while insulin goes down. The high levels of glucagon stimulate the autophagy process. That is why fasting is known as the major autophagy booster. This whole process is a form of cellular cleansing because the body first identifies substandard and old cellular equipment and marks it for destruction. The accumulation of this junk is often seen to be responsible for the effects of aging. Apart from stimulating the process of cell cleansing, fasting also stimulates the production of the growth hormone signaling the body to produce new parts for the body.

Benefits of Autophagy

Most of the research on the benefits that autophagy offers has been done in animals because of the length of time it takes. However, these benefits also apply to humans. Some of the benefits of autophagy include:

Metabolic health

Type II diabetes is often triggered by impaired autophagy. That is, when the process autophagy fails, it results in an accumulation of oxidative damage in the beta cells within the pancreas. The result is the inability to produce insulin. Autophagy protects the insulin-producing cells making autophagy a great preventative tactic that reverses pre-diabetes and keeping the blood sugar levels under control.

Healthy aging

Studies in mice and worms have found that autophagy slows down the process of aging, thus extending your lifespan dramatically. Scientists have induced autophagy in animals and found that it increased lifespan. On the contrary, when the autophagy stimulating genes were withdrawn from these animals, the lifespan boost from fasting declined, suggesting that indeed, autophagy helps in slowing aging.

Fight against cancer

A 2012 study found autophagy to be an adaptable process that selects the materials to be recycled based on the kind of stress the body is subjected to. The study further notes that autophagy plays an important role in fending off cancer, thus interfering with this process can result in malignant disease. However, other studies suggest that autophagy is a double-edged sword where cancer is concerned because it can also contribute to tumor formation. Autophagy can enhance cellular survival of cells, including cancer cells. More studies need to be done.

Heart health

A growing body of research has found that autophagy is responsible for the removal of damaged organelles and proteins in the heart cells, thus reducing the risk of heart disease and other cardiovascular diseases.

Brain health

Autophagy plays an important role in the removal of toxic proteins that often contribute to dementia. In fact, an accumulation of these proteins have been linked to the development of neurodegenerative diseases like Huntington's, Parkinson's, and Alzheimer's disease.

Other benefits of intermittent fasting include prevention of damage to the healthy tissues and organs, providing cells with molecular building blocks and energy and enhancing the immune system.

Common Myths about Intermittent Fasting

There are a lot of myths that have autophagy. Some of the common myths that you need to know about autophagy include the following:

You need to fast for 3-5 days to activate autophagy. Autophagy is a catabolic state that triggers by energy deprivation. This means that you need to induce energy deprivation to trigger autophagy and burn through the endogenous fuel of the body. While it's true that you need to fast for at three days to get your body into a state of ketosis and eventually trigger autophagy, this only applies to someone that is eating a normal diet with no calorie restriction. It's important to keep in mind that autophagy is regulated by the balance between AMPK and mTOR.

You can activate autophagy with a 24-hour fast. The truth is that it's impossible to get a significant boost of autophagy with a one day fast. You have to partner fasting with other factors that trigger autophagy like HIIT exercises. A 16-24 hour fast will not give you the most in terms of autophagy because actually, fasting doesn't begin with skipping a meal. Your body will go into the fasted state after 5-6 hours of not eating.

More autophagy is better. It's believed that you can gain more from autophagy by fasting for a minimum of three days by boosting stem cells, fighting cancers, and tumors. Well, you'll be surprised to know that more is not always better. Excessive autophagy can have negative side effects; for instance, some bacteria and parasites thrive and replicate under autophagy, and tumor cells can also have their fitness against environmental stressors enhanced. Too much autophagy can result in sarcopenia and muscle wasting that can jeopardize longevity. This means that while autophagy is amazing, it's not ideal all the time.

Autophagy is equivalent to starvation. Autophagy is not equivalent to starvation. It's easy to assume that abstaining from food makes you starve. While you're technically starving because your body is not relying on calories from food, your body isn't entirely deprived of energy. This is because your body stores some body fat that it uses for energy when you don't eat. Moreover, during autophagy, your body goes through healing and self-renewal that doesn't happen when you're eating. Thus, it's wrong to equate autophagy to starvation.

Drinking coffee hinders autophagy. Taking non-caloric coffee doesn't break your fast and subsequently autophagy. If anything, coffee is important in activating autophagy alongside ketosis. This is because of the presence of polyphenol, a compound that promotes the autophagy process. Caffeine also allows your body to embrace lipolysis, which is simply a process of burning fat, boosting AMPK and improving ketones and reducing insulin.

Autophagy Mistakes you Must Avoid

It's likely that you'd want to activate autophagy in order to tap into the many benefits it offers. This could mean making certain mistakes that are counterproductive to your efforts. Here are some of the autophagy mistakes you need to avoid:

Taking artificial sweeteners. While some artificial sweeteners purport to be calorie-free, they are bound to increase your insulin levels. When this happens, your appetite levels rise even as gastric juices are released long before you eat.

Consuming fewer food nutrients. When you fast, you must make sure that you consume sufficient amounts of nutrients during the feeding window. Failure to eat take sufficient nutrients will put your overall health in jeopardy. Therefore, be sure to include nutrient-dense foods like pastured eggs, organ meats, vegetables, fruits, and herbs, among others.

Not exercising. Although intermittent fasting by itself will activate autophagy, it needs to be combined with proper nutrition, better sleep, and exercise. Thus, be sure to incorporate low impact exercises in your intermittent fasting plan so that you get the most from the plan.

Inconsistencies in your circadian rhythm. For you to achieve autophagy, you need to go beyond mere fasting. You must also make sure you're getting adequate and restful sleep. This is because the growth hormone is also released when you're asleep. Thus, to get the most of autophagy, you need to consider going to bed early to allow for a major repair to take place.

Consuming fatty coffee. Although it's not expected that fat will raise your insulin levels as proteins and carbs do, fats raise mTOR levels putting your body in the feeding state. Therefore, it's safe to stay away from all fasts so that you don't interfere with the autophagy process.

Taking supplements with calories. Some calories come with extra sugar and calories. While they may be safe to use, you must look out for their caloric content so that you don't up piling calories that will eventually break your fast.

Autophagy cleans out your cells, making them new. Science has proven that this process can be activated by fasting, exercise and other supplements will increase autophagy, helping you to age better, build a stronger brain, and stay better. However, you must pay attention to the different things that are likely to hinder autophagy so that you get the most out of your intermittent fasting and autophagy.

Chapter 6: Intermittent Fasting of Techniques

As the intermittent fasting phenomenon continues to sweep across the weight loss and wellness world, it's important to understand that there are many different approaches to intermittent fasting. Whichever method of fasting you'll settle for is all a matter of preference. Here is an overview of some of the intermittent fasting methods:

Eat Stop Eat (5/2 Diet)

This method of fasting was advanced by Brad Pilon but popularized by Michael Mosley, a British journalist. It's the most popular of the intermittent fasting protocols. This fasting method requires you to fast for 24 hours so that you're only having dinner for two days in a week. This method of fasting aims to impose a bigger caloric deficit on the days when you're fasting. This means that you shouldn't overeat because this will beat logic and lead to weight gain. You, however, get to eat normally on the remaining five days of the week. This diet doesn't have restrictions on the kinds of food you should eat; thus, most people find it easy to stick to compared to traditional diets.

How to Do the 5/2 Diet

With this diet, you get to eat normally for five days a week without any calorie restriction. However, you get to restrict your calorie intake to between 500 and 600 per day for two days. You're at liberty to choose the days of the week when you fast and when you'll eat normally. Most people prefer to fast on Mondays and Thursdays and normally eat for the remainder of the days. Even then, keep in mind that eating normally doesn't amount to eating anything, especially junk food, because this will certainly hamper your weight loss goals. The secret is eating the same amount of food you'd eat if you weren't fasting.

The eat stop eat diet is quite effective for weight loss when done well. The reason is simple; this eating plan lets you consume fewer calories. As such, you shouldn't try to compensate for the days you're fasting by eating too much on your non-fasting days. The interesting thing about this intermittent fasting method is that it doesn't define when or what you should eat on the days you are fasting. Whether you want to begin the day with breakfast or start eating later in the day, make sure you don't exceed the 500-600 calories. This means that you can have three small meals or two slightly bigger meals. Some of the food options with less caloric content but leave you feeling full include vegetables, natural yogurt with berries, baked/boiled eggs, grilled fish, cauliflower rice, low-calorie soup, water and tea among others. While intermittent fasting is generally safe, you need to avoid this method of fasting it if you have a history of eating disorders, you often experience a drop in blood sugar levels, you're trying to conceive or are malnourished.

The 16:8 Intermittent Fasting Method

The 16:8 intermittent fasting method involves voluntary abstinence from food for at least 16 hours so that your hours of eating are limited to the eight per day. However, you may consume non-caloric drinks like water during the 16 hours of fasting. You're free to determine the frequency of your fast. It's a matter of preference, depending on whether you want to stay healthy or lose weight and fat. Unlike diets that often have strict regulations, this method of fasting is easy to follow, yet it provides real results. 16:8 is less restrictive and more flexible compared to most of the diet plans. This makes it easy to fit into any lifestyle easily.

Getting Started with the 16:8 Diet

To get started with the 16:8 intermittent fasting method, you need to identify an eight-hour window during which you will eat. It's common to find most people eating between noon and eight pm because you only get to fast overnight and skip breakfast which is manageable. You may also want to consider eating between 9 am and 5 pm, giving you time for a healthy breakfast. No matter the time you select, make sure it fits into your schedule perfectly. It's advisable to eat a number of small meals spaced through the day. This is critical in stabilizing blood sugar and keeping hunger under control. Most importantly, sticking to nutritious whole foods will help in maximizing the potential health benefits of your diet. Including nutrient-dense foods in your diet lets you reap the benefits of this regimen. Some of the best food options include fruits such as apples, berries, and oranges, vegetables like cauliflower, broccoli and tomatoes, whole grains that include rice, oats, quinoa and barley, healthy fats like avocadoes and coconut oil and various sources of proteins that include eggs, legumes, poultry, meat and seeds. The 16:8 intermittent fasting method is quite popular because it's flexible, convenient, easy to follow, and sustainable over time.

Drawbacks of 16:8

Although this intermittent fasting plan offers numerous benefits, it's not short of drawbacks. Having an 8-hour feeding window can come with the temptation to eat more than they normally would to make up for the extended hours without food. As a result, you may end up gaining weight, developing poor eating habits, or even experiencing digestive problems. You could also experience short term negative side effects like fatigue, hunger, and weakness. However, these will subside when you get used to the routine. While these are common and expected, be sure to seek professional health when the effects seem to get out of hand. It's advisable that you talk to your doctor before giving this fasting method a try, particularly if you have a prevailing health condition.

Alternate Day Fasting

This intermittent fasting method allows you to fast every alternate day. However, you can eat just about everything on the days when you're not fasting. This method of fasting is powerful and has been linked to lowering the risk of heart diseases as well as type 2 diabetes.

How to Do Alternate Day Fasting

The idea behind alternate day fasting is that you fast one day and skip the next day. This means that you'll be restricting what you eat half the time. On the days when you're fasting, you can drink as much of the calorie-free drinks and beverages as you like. These include unsweetened tea and coffee, and water. You can also modify this intermittent fasting approach to consume at least 500 calories on the days when you're fasting. This is because the weight loss benefits will still be the same. Alternate day fasting is thus more appealing for many people than the traditional everyday restriction of calories. Studies have shown that you can lose up to 8% of your body weight with alternate-day fasting within a period of 2-12 weeks. More specifically, this method of fasting coupled with daily calorie restriction is usually effective in reducing harmful belly fat as well as other inflammatory markers, especially in people who are obese.

A review study conducted in 2016 concluded that alternate day fasting could be superior to the daily calorie restriction because of the fact that it's easier to stick to, preserves more muscle mass and produces greater fat loss. Moreover, when combined with endurance exercises, alternate-day fasting can result in twice as much weight loss than Alternate Day Fasting alone, and six times as much weight loss as endurance exercise alone. Interestingly, this fasting protocol is equally effective when done alongside a low fat or high-fat diet.

Alternate Day Fasting and Hunger

It's worth noting that alternate day fasting has inconsistencies when it comes to hunger. While some studies have concluded that hunger will go down, others suggest that hunger is unchanged. Even then, it's been concluded that this method of fasting is way better and tolerable compared to going on a full fast. One study showed that this method of fasting resulted in changes in the hunger hormone (ghrelin) as well as the satiety hormone (leptin). Similarly, modified forms of this intermittent fasting decreased the number of hunger hormones while increasing the satiety hormones being produced.

Alternate day fasting is particularly instrumental in improving or reversing the symptoms of type 2 diabetes. This mode of fasting causes mild reductions in the risk factors for type 2 diabetes in obese and overweight people. Alternate day fasting is even more effective in reducing insulin resistance and lowering insulin levels while demonstrating a slight effect in the control of blood sugar. This eventually leads to a reduced risk of type 2 diabetes. On the other hand, the loss of weight in obese and overweight individuals reduces the risk of heart disease and related conditions.

The Warrior Diet

The warrior diet is a unique mode of fasting because it cycles between extended periods of taking little food and short windows of overeating. This method of fasting has been found to be effective in losing weight and improving energy levels as well as promoting mental clarity. It mimics the early warriors who ate very little food during the day but fasted during the night. It was created by Ori Hofmekler, a former member of the Israeli Special Forces in 2001. This method of fasting was designed to improve the way we eat, perform, feel, and look by placing emphasis on the body through a reduced intake of food, eventually triggering survival instincts. This method of fasting is based on personal beliefs, not science. When you follow this diet, you'll be undereating during the 20 hours of fasting but can binge on any foods within the 4hour feeding window. Even then, it's encouraged that you mostly focus on eating healthy, organic, and unprocessed foods. This method of fasting has proven to contribute to fat burning, boosting energy levels, improving concentration, and stimulating cellular repair.

Potential Pitfalls of the Warrior Diet

Besides the benefits of following the warrior diet, this pattern of eating presents some pitfalls that include the following:

It's inappropriate for people. People suffering from heart failure, type 1 diabetes, and certain types of cancers should not practice this pattern of eating. The same goes for people with a history of eating disorders, expectant women, and extreme athletes.

It's likely to end up in disordered eating. This method of fasting emphasizes on overeating during the four-hour feeding window. This can be problematic for some people even though the creator insists that you should be able to tell when to stop eating. Binging on large quantities of food may also result in feelings of shame and regret that can have a negative impact on your mental health.

It could lead to negative side effects. The warrior diet can present some unpleasant side effects that include dizziness, fatigue, light-headedness, insomnia, extreme hunger, constipation, low blood sugar, irritability, and hormonal imbalance, among others. Additionally, health professionals hold the opinion that you can also be deprived of nutrients. Even then, you can strive to ensure that you're eating nutrient-dense foods at all times.

How to Do the Warrior Diet

According to Hofmekler, you need to execute the warrior diet in three phases in order to improve your body's ability to utilize fat as energy as follows:

Phase 1 – Detox. You will be undereating for 20 hours by including the following food choices; clear broth, vegetable juices, hard-boiled eggs, raw fruits, dairy, and vegetables. You can then eat a salad with vinegar and oil dressing for the next hour followed by one large meal with plant-based proteins, small amounts of cheese, wheat-free whole grains, and cooked vegetables. You're free to consume tea, water, and coffee throughout the day. This phase lasts for one week.

Phase 2 – High Fat. You will still be undereating for 20 hours by including the following food choices; clear broth, vegetable juices, hard-boiled eggs, raw fruits, dairy, and vegetables. However, during the overrating period, you will include a lean animal protein, cooked vegetables, a handful of nuts, and a salad with vinegar and oil dressing. Don't consume any starches or grains in this phase. This phase also lasts for one week.

Phase 3 – Concluding Fat Loss. This period alternates between periods of consuming high carb and low protein. That is, you have 1-2 days of taking high carbs, followed by another 1-2 days of high protein and low carbs. During the high carb days, you will under-eat during the 20 hours of fasting on vegetable juices, dairy, broth, hard-boiled eggs, and raw fruits. You can then eat an oil and vinegar dressing vegetable salad, small amounts of animal protein, and one main carbohydrate during the overeating period.

On the high protein and low carb days, under-eat during the 20 hours of fasting on vegetable juices, dairy, broth, hard-boiled eggs, and raw fruits. However, when it comes to the overeating period, you'll eat an oil and vinegar dressing vegetable salad, an animal protein of between 8-16 ounces and non-starchy vegetables. While you shouldn't consume grains and starches in this phase, you can also eat a small amount of fresh tropical fruit as a dessert.

48-Hour Fast

A 48-hour fast is the longest duration that you can practice with intermittent fasting. Most intermittent fasting protocols cover shorter durations. Therefore, if you opt to go for this fast, you need to be well informed so that you take the drawbacks into consideration.

Doing a 48-Hour Fast

The 48-hour fast means that you don't eat anything over a period of two full days. For example, if you stop eating after dinner on the first day, you will eat again at the same time on the third day. You're at liberty to drink zero-calorie drinks and water during the fasting period. Taking the length of the fasting window into account, you must make sure you're taking plenty of fluids so that you're well hydrated. And when you get to your eating window, make sure you're reintroducing food gradually so that you don't overstimulate your gut resulting diarrhea, nausea and bloating. You should have a light first post past snack like a handful of almonds followed by another small meal an hour or two later. You can do a 48-hour first once or twice a month as opposed to weekly. This ensures that you derive greater health benefits from the fast.

Drawbacks of 48-Hour Fasting

There are a number of downsides linked to doing a 48-hour fast. To begin with, this intermittent fasting method is not suitable for everyone, thus the longer you fast, the greater the side effects. Some of the common side effects to look out for include:

Sluggishness and exhaustion. During the first 24 hours of fasting, you will experience a drop in the stored carbs forcing the body to burn fat for energy. This may result in a feeling of sluggishness and exhaustion after 24 hours, especially if you're fasting for this long for the first time. This method of fasting is more difficult to stick to because of the extended duration of fasting. Therefore, you may want to start with a shorter fast and progress over time.

Dizziness and hunger. One of the main drawbacks of 48-hour fasting is severe hunger even though this is mostly temporary. In one study involving 768 people fasting for 48 hours, 72% of the participants experienced fatigue, hunger, dizziness, and insomnia.

Interference with social eating. Most types of fasting often interfere with your social eating so that you're not able to go out to meals with family and friends. Yet food is a major aspect to most cultural practices. This means that you need to consider if you're willing to give up your social eating for the fast.

It's risky for some populations. Although the whole idea behind practicing intermittent fasting is to enjoy the benefits it promises, it poses a risk for some people such as people with type 1 diabetes, people with low blood pressure, women who have a history of amenorrhea or are trying to conceive, those who are taking certain medications and people who are underweight.

Minimizing the Side Effects of 48-Hour Fasting

Some of the common side effects that the 48-hour fast presents can be prevented with the right measures. Fasting for a lengthy period can result in dehydration if you don't take enough fluids or consume enough electrolytes manly magnesium, sodium, calcium, and potassium that are depleted when you abstain from food.

Here are some tips to prevent complications during fasting:

- Drink unsweetened black coffee or green tea to help in managing hunger levels.
- Stay hydrated by drinking plenty of water with a pinch of salt or electrolyte tablets.
- Occupy yourself with numerous activities so that you are not obsessed with hunger. You can watch a movie, take a walk or listen to a podcast, among other things.

Overall, the 48-hour fast offers a number of benefits that include weight loss, cell repair, and heightened insulin sensitivity.

Spontaneous Meal Skipping

You don't have to follow through a well-structured intermittent fasting plan for you to experience the benefits of fasting. You can actually skip meals spontaneously from time to time when you are too busy to cook or are not hungry. The human body is well conditioned to stay for lengthy periods so you can skip a meal a day when you're really not hungry and eat the next meal. This also goes when you're traveling and can't find anything to eat. Skipping a meal or 2 when you feel inclined is basically a form of spontaneous fast that will get you results over time.

To sum it all up, intermittent fasting is not everyone's cup of tea. So, you shouldn't put too much pressure on yourself when one or all of these intermittent fasting methods don't seem to work for you. Make sure that you evaluate the benefits you're getting from fasting against the setbacks so before proceeding with a plan or abandoning it altogether.

Chapter 7: Tips for a Smooth Transition into Intermittent Fasting

It's common to hear stories of women who started intermittent fasting but quit long before they settled in the routine. The reason for this is often because they started it all wrong. The manner in which you ease into intermittent fasting will determine whether your experience will be a success or not. So how do you transition into intermittent fasting? Here are some tips to help you get started:

Talk to your doctor

It's important that you talk to your doctor before starting on any of the intermittent fasting protocols. This is especially important if you have a medical condition or are feeling unwell. The doctor is in a position to offer you sound advice to help you pull through or abandon the idea altogether.

Find a suitable intermittent fasting method

While all the intermittent fasting offers various benefits, you need to know that not all the methods are suitable for everyone. Moreover, not every intermittent fasting protocol will help you to achieve your goal. So, take time to understand the different methods of fasting and their subsequent benefits to determine what will work for you. Most importantly, you need to opt for a plan that you can follow with ease.

Start with a few hour fasts

It's impractical to jump into a 16 hour fast when you're used to eating 5-6 times a day. You need to get your body to embrace the new pattern of eating by beginning with fewer hours of fasting advancing gradually until you get to the point where you can fast for 16 hours. You can begin with a 12 hour fast, gradually reducing the hours you're eating as you get comfortable with the process.

Eat normally at first

It can be confusing when you have multiple changes taking place at the same time. In fact, in such cases, you're likely to give up on your intermittent fasting experience. Thus, instead of overhauling your entire diet at the time you're beginning intermittent fasting do it gradually. Begin by introducing healthier food options into your diet alongside a few hours of fasting. Once you have gotten used to clean eating and are eating normally, then you can focus on extending your hours of fasting to fit the intermittent fasting plan you're aiming to follow.

Have a protein-filled breakfast

By now, it's obvious that breakfast is not actually the most important meal of the day. However, if you opt to have breakfast, make sure that it is rich in proteins. A breakfast meal that is protein-rich will give you a satiating feeling for most of the day so that you don't have the temptation to sneak in snacks along the way. Moreover, your blood sugar levels will be more stable. This way, you'll find it pretty easy to stick to the intermittent fasting plan you have chosen.

Drink plenty of fluids to stay hydrated

Both hunger and thirst are processed by the same part of the brain. As such, oftentimes what we interpret as hunger is usually thirst. Therefore, you end up eating even when you don't really have to. Therefore, it's important to make sure you hydrate well when you wake up, especially if you're not going to eat breakfast. Proper hydration is the key to keeping hydration pangs at bay, so you don't have to think you're hungry when you're actually not.

Eat high fat and carb-rich meals at night

This may seem counterproductive. However, the reality is that you can't give up carbs entirely. Instead, you can have them at night to increase your blood sugar levels at night so that it takes time before it falls since you will be adding fat and protein. This means that when your blood sugar levels fall, you will be asleep.

Having carbs also increases the production of serotonin, leaving you feeling great after your meal so that you don't want to eat anymore.

Switch up your timings to fit into your lifestyle

It's important to remember that the intermittent fasting schedule should work for you and not the other way around. Therefore, work around a plan that accommodates your lifestyle in terms of when you can comfortably eat without interfering with your work schedule and other responsibilities. When you're flexible with your fasting hours, you can be sure to create a workable approach.

Stick to your fasting and feasting window

When you start off on an intermittent fasting method with defined hours of eating and feasting, make sure that you don't keep on changing. This is the reason why it's usually hard for most people to ease into intermittent fasting. When you keep on changing your timings, you eventually confuse the body because what you'll be doing is reprogramming your hunger cues.

Have a mantra to keep you going

The truth is that it'll take time before your body can get accustomed to the intermittent fasting method of your choice. As a matter of fact, intermittent fasting will come down to strengthening your willpower. When you have words of encouragement to keep you going, it will empower you to get through the tough times when you feel like giving up no matter the time of day.

Keep yourself busy

The fact that you're fasting is not a reason to also be idle. Instead, pay attention to your day to day activities so that you don't obsess about fasting and how hungry you will or are feeling. Make sure you keep yourself busy. This may mean leaving the house to run errands, attending meetings, or even taking a walk.

Keep off social media before bed

Social media is a gateway to a whole lot of information. It's here that your friends can share their favorite recipes and you can be tempted after seeing them. In fact, even if you were not thinking about anything, you might want to eat after seeing some of those pictures.

Lower your expectations

You must understand that it took months and in some cases, years of eating ice cream, chocolate, pizza, and more to put on weight. Now you don't expect to lose weight instantly. That will be too ambitious. It will take time before you can begin noticing a change.

Focus on your purpose

It's important to keep in mind the reason why you're getting into intermittent fasting in the first place. If your goal is weight loss or weight maintenance, longevity, and relieving symptoms of certain diseases, you will focus on achieving this goal whenever you feel like giving up.

Address your worries.

It' advisable that you address any issues that may make you nervous so that you stop intermittent fasting. For instance, it's okay to skip breakfast contrary to what most health and fitness experts' advice. It's also okay to avoid snacks because snacking will not help you lose weight. Most importantly, your metabolism will not slow down when you fast. If anything, intermittent fasting will increase your metabolism and help you to retain more muscle while you lose weight.

Choose nutrient-dense foods

You need to eat foods that are high in fiber, minerals, vitamins as well as other nutrients. This helps in keeping your blood sugar levels steady and prevent nutrient deficiencies. Having a balanced diet also contributes to weight loss and overall health.

Keep track of your progress

You will do well to keep a journal of your thoughts and how you feel physically and emotionally so that you're able to tell the progress you are making. Where possible, take photos at the beginning of the journey and make comparisons with subsequent photos to determine the change your body is going through.

Stay away from food

When you're fasting, it's reasonable that you stay away from food to fend off the temptation to eat. This may mean avoiding shopping when your fasting, walking past your favorite bakery, attending your best friend's birthday, or preparing food for other people who are not fasting. The reason for this is simple; you can't eat what you don't see.

Understand your calorie needs

It's unrealistic to get into intermittent fasting without knowing your calorie needs. If your goal is to lose weight, then you need to consider a plan that will help in creating a calorie deficit. This means that you will need to consume fewer calories than your body is burning.

Create a meal plan

Although intermittent fasting is not strict in terms of the foods you should eat, having a meal plan is a great way to help you stay focused. A meal plan will also help you to stay away from the temptation of eating foods that are likely to be a hindrance to achieving your goals. When you plan your meals, it also ensures that you include all the nutrients you need.

Don't give in to the temptation to overeat

Going for a few more hours without food as you're used to is not easy. Thus, you may naturally have the temptation to eat too much when the time to eat comes. You can avoid this temptation by making sure you are well hydrated throughout the day.

Exercise in the evenings

Working out in the morning means you have to wake up early. As a result, you'll have more hours of going without food. Thus, you can turn things around so that instead of waking up early to work out, you do post-dinner workouts. Working out will reduce your hunger temporarily by raising the levels of peptide, the hormone that is responsible for suppressing appetite. Although you will be tired, working out before going to bed will leave you feeling satisfied even though tired.

Brush your teeth after dinner

Brushing your teeth is a great bedtime cue that helps to switch your mind from food. When you brush your teeth, you are communicating to your body that you are done with eating for the day.

Limit your intake of white carbs

This may seem like a contradiction, especially because intermittent fasting is not a diet per se but a pattern of eating. Eating white carbs like bread and rice will raise your blood sugar levels. This will then dip faster and leave you feeling cranky and hungry. So, don't use intermittent fasting as an excuse to indulge in cake instead, strive to balance the good carbs with fat and proteins to avoid experiencing extreme hunger.

Chapter 8: Common Intermittent Fasting Myths

Although there's a lot of information on the internet about intermittent fasting, not everything you've heard about this pattern of eating is true. This chapter set the record straight about some of the common intermittent fasting myths:

Intermittent fasting will make you overeat

Some people claim that intermittent fasting makes you overeat during the feasting window. While you may have a large meal than usual to compensate for the calories lost during fasting, you'll hardly go beyond the compensation level. One study found that those who fasted ate only 500 more calories compared to more than 2,400 calories they had missed while fasting. Due to the reduced food intake and declining insulin levels, while boosting metabolism, human growth hormone (HGH) levels, and norepinephrine levels, intermittent fasting will make you lose fat. One review observed that fasting for 3-24 weeks led to a 4-7% belly loss and 3-8% weight loss.

Intermittent fasting is bad for your health

Although you may have heard that intermittent fasting is bad for your health, studies have found such impressive health benefits.

For instance, intermittent fasting will bring about a change in gene expression related to immunity and longevity. In fact, fasting has been found to prolong lifespan among animals. Additionally, fasting also has major metabolic benefits like a reduction in the level of oxidative stress, heart disease risk, and inflammation. Fasting may also boost your brain health through the elevation of brain-derived neurotrophic factor (BDNF), which is a hormone that helps in protecting you against mental conditions such as depression.

Intermittent fasting will make you lose muscle

Some people hold the belief that by fasting, you lose muscle as your body relies on muscle for fuel. Although this is a common occurrence during dieting, there is no concrete evidence linking fasting to more muscle loss compared to other diets. Instead, studies have shown that intermittent fasting is a far much better option when it comes to maintaining muscle mass. One review showed that fasting had the same amount of weight loss as calorie restriction even though the reduction in muscle mass was far much less. Yet another study showed a slight increase in muscle mass in individuals who ate all their calories in one large meal in the evening. Even more interesting is the fact that intermittent fasting is popular among bodybuilders who have found it to help in maintaining their muscle along with low body percentage. There's no conclusive evidence linking fasting to muscle loss.

You need to eat often to maximize muscle gain. Some people hold that your body is able to digest only 30 grams of protein per meal, meaning you need to eat every after a short interval to maximize muscle gain. Unfortunately, this claim is not backed by science. If anything, studies have shown that when you eat your protein in more frequent doses, it doesn't have an effect on your muscle mass. Rather the most important factor to consider is the overall amount of protein you've consumed.

Intermittent fasting will put the body in starvation mode

A popular argument about intermittent fasting is that it's capable of putting your body in starvation mode so that your metabolism is shut; thus, you can't burn fat. This is actually laughable because starvation is on the extreme. Although it's true that when you lose weight in the long term, it'll reduce the number of calories you burn with time, this is the expected result no matter the weight-loss approach you take. There's no evidence linking intermittent fasting to a greater decline in the number of calories burned compared to the other weight-loss strategies. Short term fasts will increase your metabolic rate because of the drastic increase in the level of norepinephrine in the blood that stimulates metabolism and signals the fat cells to break down body fat. Studies have found that doing a 48-hour fast will boost your metabolism by 3.6-14%. Even then, fasting for a longer period than this can reverse these effects resulting in decreased metabolism. One study found that fasting for 22 days every other day didn't result in a decline in the metabolic rate but a 4% loss in fat mass.

It's healthy to eat every often

Some people are convinced that eating often is good for your health. Even then, this position overlooks the benefits of short term fasting to cellular repair processes like autophagy during which cells utilize the old and dysfunctional proteins for their energy. The process of autophagy helps the body to fight against cancer as well as neurodegenerative conditions like Alzheimer's disease. This shows that occasional fasting is actually beneficial for your metabolic health. Interestingly, some studies have shown that eating or snacking often will harm your health in addition to raising your risk of disease. For instance, a study found that eating a high-calorie diet with several meals resulted in a substantial increase in fat in the liver, which is a risk factor for fatty liver disease. Observational studies have also shown that people who eat often usually have a higher risk of colorectal cancer.

Your brain requires a regular supply of glucose

It's claimed that not eating carbs after every few hours will result in your brain not functioning because your brain needs glucose as fuel. The reality is that your body has stored energy and is capable of producing the glucose that is needed through gluconeogenesis. Moreover, your body is still able to produce ketone bodies from dietary fats during a very low carb diet, starvation, and fasting. These ketone bodies then feed parts of your brain, thereby reducing the glucose requirement significantly. However, if you experience fatigue or even feel shaky when you fast, then consider frequently snacking, albeit while you pay attention to your calorie intake.

Having frequent meals helps in weight loss

The proponents of this ride on the fact that eating frequently will give your metabolism a boost. Well, not that you know it doesn't, eating frequently doesn't have an impact on your weight loss quest either. A study done on 16 obese adults comparing the effects of having three meals and six meals daily found no difference in loss of appetite or weight. Eating more often will usually make it difficult for you to adapt to any diet. Even then, if eating small meals often will help you consume less junk and fewer calories then, stick by it.

When you eat frequently, you reduce hunger

Some people believe that eating more often is a great way to deal with excessive hunger and prevent cravings. Well, the evidence for this is mixed. While some studies suggest that eating meals frequently will lead to reduced hunger, other studies have found there was no effect, and in others, the hunger levels increased. A study that compared eating three to six high protein meals per day found that eating three meals reduced hunger effectively. Ultimately, the response is dependent on the individual. Even then, there's no sufficient evidence to prove that eating more often and snacking frequently reduces hunger for everyone.

Fasting frequently will boost your metabolism

Most people believe that eating frequently will increase your metabolic rate making your body to burn more calories overall. The truth is that your body uses some calories during digestion in what is known as the thermic effect of food (TEF). This process uses about 10% of your total calorie intake. Even then, the most important thing is the number of calories you consume as opposed to the number of meals you eat. You'll be surprised that consuming 500 calories in a meal has the same effect as consuming a 100-calorie meal taking into account the 10% TEF you'll burn in both cases. Thus, whether you increase or decrease, your meal frequency will not affect the number of calories you burn.

Skipping breakfast will make you fat

This is informed by the popular belief that breakfast is the most important meal of the day. People believe that when you skip breakfast, you'll experience cravings and excessive hunger leading up to excessive weight gain. A study done among 283 adults who were overweight and obese found no difference between those who ate breakfast and those who skipped. This means that breakfast doesn't really have an effect on your weight even though there may be some individual variability. Breakfast may be beneficial for people and not others, especially those who record negative consequences.

You'll lose weight with intermittent fasting, no matter what

One of the reasons why intermittent fasting has gained popularity, especially among women is because of its promise of weight loss. Even then, you need to know that it's not automatic that when you fast, you must lose weight. This is a misconception because the process of weight loss involves a number of factors. For instance, if you fast for extended periods but eat unhealthy foods like candy and pizza when you break your fast, then chances are you'll not experience a drop in your weight. The same goes for exercising. This means that as you fast, you also must take into account other significant factors to attain your weight loss goal.

You can binge eat during your feasting window

If you have attempted intermittent fasting, then you'll know that it's common to always look forward to the feasting period when you get to throw down. This is not the time to binge eat rather stay disciplined and eat as you'd normally do, only that you emphasize on including healthy food choices in your diet. When you overeat during the feasting window, it's absolutely counterproductive because it will negate to all the work you may have put in fasting.

You can't work out when you're fasting

Most people consider working out while fasting to be a negative thing. The truth is that it's actually a positive thing as it complements your fitness efforts. Some fitness experts suggest that it's best to work out on an empty stomach. This is because you'll be burning fat that is stored in your body, thus resulting in weight loss as opposed to expending the energy from the food you just consumed. Even then, be sure to eat after working out so as to replenish your body.

Fasting to lose weight is far much better compared to the other weight-loss strategies

The popularity of intermittent fasting has made many people think that it's as easy as an on/off button when compared to other weight loss methods. The reality is that intermittent fasting requires discipline and commitment without which you will not achieve any tangible results. In fact, you can only achieve results with intermittent fasting when you do it right.

Intermittent fasting will make you fit and healthy

When combined with a proper exercise regimen, intermittent fasting can assist your weight loss efforts. Even then, you must realize that this is not a magical approach. You have to work towards achieving your goal and not taking anything for granted. Fasting alone will not give you the ideal body you desire overnight. Furthermore, once you lose weight, you have to keep on working to maintain a healthy lifestyle that includes eating nutritious meals and exercising regularly.

All intermittent fasting methods are the same, and will give everyone the same results

As discussed earlier, intermittent fasting methods differ from each other in many ways. Consequently, these methods offer different benefits to different people. Therefore, don't fall into the temptation of comparing yourself to other people who are intermittent fasting, especially when you're not getting the same results they're getting.

Chapter 9: Mistakes to Avoid During Intermittent Fasting

You may have already heard about the benefits of intermittent fasting that have propelled this eating pattern to popularity. If you've decided to try this method of eating but can't see any results yet, it may be that you're doing it wrong. There are certain mistakes you can inadvertently make that will make this experience difficult. Here are some common mistakes you need to avoid to make your intermittent fasting journey a success:

Making radical changes to your routine. Making a turnaround from a 3-4 hour eating intervals to an 8-hour eating window can be challenging. This is because you're likely to feel hungry all the time. This can be discouraging. In fact, some people quit their intermittent fasting attempt at this point before their bodies even get to adjust from their regular eating pattern. Generally, it may take up to 10 days before you can settle into your new eating pattern and stop feeling hungry during the fasting window. To help you to transition smoothly, begin by stretching out the number of hours between meals until you are able to attain a 12-hour fasting window comfortably. You can then build on this to at least 16 hours of fasting and 8 hours of eating.

Putting fasting at the center of your life. When you start on intermittent fasting, you're likely to wrap your mind and thoughts around intermittent fasting. You may find that you're opting out of dinner with family or turning down invitations to parties because you're on a fast. This generally makes intermittent fasting unsustainable and less enjoyable in the long run. Instead, consider working on an intermittent fasting schedule that fits into your lifestyle and schedule so that you can comfortably accommodate your social events. After all, intermittent fasting isn't a diet that spells out what you should eat.

Overeating during your eating window. When you start fasting, overeating can be easy when the fast ends. This may be triggered by the attempt to justify yourself that you need to make up for lost calories or you're just feeling ravenous. This is not a good approach, especially if you're fasting to achieve weight loss. Moreover, overeating after an extended fast could result in a number of problems like stomach aches and diarrhea, among others. Therefore, you'll do well to have a meal plan that serves as a guide so that you are able to prepare a healthy meal as your fast comes to an end. Aim at using whole ingredients like plenty of vegetables, lean protein, and whole grains wherever possible.

Giving up too soon. Although it sounds theoretically simple, the intermittent fasting pattern of eating is not easy to follow. This pattern of eating automatically cuts on your calories by shortening your eating window so that you're running on fewer calories. This means that not every plan will work for you, depending on your lifestyle. Therefore, rather than give up be patient or try a different fasting method other than the one you have started with until you find what works for you.

Lack of exercise/activity. It's common to have a pre-workout snack before hitting the gym. As such, entertaining the thought of working our while you're fasting may be foreign. If you're thinking along these lines, then it's important to remember that your body will always have adequate energy that it stores as fat for use when you don't feed for a reasonable period. Even then, it's always important to consult your doctor just to be sure that it is safe to exercise while fasting. Otherwise, you can continue with your usual workout routine or even try some low impact exercises like walking. If you fast overnight and exercise, make sure you eat a protein-rich meal to increase the rate at which you will build muscle.

Drinking wrong liquids. It's important to make sure that you stay hydrated during fasting so that you don't feel week or excessively hungry. You can drink water, tea, and coffee throughout the day. However, tea and coffee shouldn't be sweetened. The idea is to avoid any calorie-filled or protein-filled drinks and beverages since they will affect your insulin levels and are capable of halting autophagy that you are actually seeking to promote. This means that you need to keep off diet sodas as well as anything that is sweetened heavily. Remember that some zero-calorie sweeteners may still have an effect on your insulin levels and stimulate the appetite. If you're finding it difficult to drink up, you can use apps that help you to track your hydration so that you're sticking to water, coffee, and tea all day long.

Eating unhealthy food. Although intermittent fasting mainly focuses on when you eat while overlooking at the quality of food you eat, you must strive to eat healthy foods, especially if you want to lose weight. For instance, if you mainly eat processed foods and ignore whole foods that make up a well-balanced diet, you will have trouble achieving your health goal. Make an effort to gradually change your diet as you adjust to your new eating schedule to include healthier options. This way, you'll not be trying to overhaul everything at the same time, thus making your plan sustainable.

Choosing the wrong intermittent fasting method. You need to set yourself up for success by selecting an intermittent fasting protocol that is in line with your lifestyle and goals you are seeking to achieve. Selecting an intermittent fasting plan that is in contradiction with your lifestyle will definitely result in failure even before you get started with it. Keep in mind important aspects of life that are likely to be affected when you fast like work, your social life, and health goals.

Eating too little during your fasting window. When you're too ambitious about weight loss, you may be tempted to eat too little during your eating window despite fasting for extended durations. This is counterproductive because failure to eat enough food could actually result in weight gain. Here's why; eating too little results in the cannibalization of your muscle mass effectively slowing down metabolism. Lack of sufficient metabolic muscle mass could sabotage your ability to maintain or lose fat in the future. This is further compounded by the fact that intermittent fasting is based on arbitrary temporary rules as opposed to the real cues from the body.

You're overemphasizing on when you eat at the expense of what you eat. The main difference between intermittent fasting and other diets is that it's mainly time centered while remaining silent on what to eat. As such, you can easily fall into the trap of eating foods that are unhealthy and end up undoing the benefits of fasting. Foods and drinks like milkshake and beer will definitely stall your efforts, especially when not consumed in moderation. Remember, fasting is not magic since its benefits are based on the fact that by reducing the hours of eating, you also get to reduce the number of calories you consume.

Doing too many things at the same time. If you have made a raft of decisions aimed at turning your lifestyle around, then you should try not to implement them all at the same time. For instance, don't change your diet, over train and fast at the same time. This is akin to biting more than you can chew. Therefore, implement the changes gradually so that you're not beginning with daily training, extended fasting, and restricting calories all at the same time. This can only lead to problems because while your body is able to thrive under a little stress, too much stress is not good.

Obsessing over timings. One of the things that intermittent fasting does is helping your body to be in tune with real hunger. This is because most of the time, what we perceive to be hunger is actually thirst. Real hunger will often occur within 16-24 hours and not every four hours. You should let the body dictate when you should eat as opposed to thinking about when you will eat or even eating around the clock. If you keep on counting the hours until you can eat, your body will not understand the true hunger signals.

Feeling guilty for eating outside your feeding window. One of the important things about intermittent fasting that most people forget is the importance of listening to your body, especially if you're just starting out. If you feel too hungry and can no longer sustain a fast, it's okay to eat. When you ignore the hunger cues, you are likely to develop an unhealthy relationship with food so that you start feeling guilty whenever you have to eat outside the feeding window. This is dangerous because it can eventually result in an eating disorder.

For you to succeed in intermittent fasting, you need to make sure that you're executing it the right way. This means finding the right plan, having the right motivation, and listening to your body, among others. Most importantly pay attention to your habits to make sure that you're only embracing healthy habits. Don't just jump into the intermittent fasting craze just because everyone else is doing it but because you are keen about making a lifestyle change. The best thing to do is to make sure that you research on this pattern of eating extensively so that you're well informed when you transition into it.

Chapter 10: The Negative Effects of Intermittent Fasting

Intermittent fasting has continued to receive massive publicity that mainly focuses on the benefits of embracing this lifestyle. But have you stopped to think about the negative effects? Well, like any other diet, intermittent fasting also presents potential negative effects that you need to be aware of before getting into it so that you make informed choices. Here are some of the negative effects of intermittent fasting; you need to know before you try the trendy diet plan:

You'll experience real hunger. If you're used to eating every so often throughout the day, then you will have problems with intermittent fasting because you'll experience real hunger. When this happens, you shouldn't give up right away and break your fast. Instead, take active steps to help you to keep going. For instance, you need to make sure you stay away from food, including the smell of food as these can distract you and trigger the release of gastric acid in your stomach, making you feel hungry. You'll also do well to make sure you're well-hydrated in addition to distracting yourself by reading a book, going to the movie or going on a walk.

Intermittent fasting has risks. A lot of what is said about intermittent fasting are the benefits. But you will be surprised to learn that there are risks linked to this pattern of eating. That is why you need to begin by having a conversation with your doctor, especially if you're more than 65 years old and at risk of health complications. Intermittent fasting also puts you at risk if your job involves lifting heavy equipment because you could experience low blood sugar and light-headedness that could endanger the lives of others. Other categories of people who are at risk and must top fasting immediately include those who are underweight, pregnant, have diabetes, are taking medications, have a history of amenorrhea, are breastfeeding, have an eating disorder, you are struggling with perfectionism or have mood instability.

Infertility. You need sufficient nutrient intake to make sure that your reproductive health is well sustained. This is especially true of amenorrhea that is directly linked to low body weight and under-eating. Although not so many studies have been done on human beings, intermittent fasting is restrictive in nature and is likely to interfere with nature. A study on rats established that intermittent fasting interfered with fertility in rats.

Intermittent fasting could result in disordered eating. Although there is little documentation of intermittent fasting in humans, this pattern of eating is likely to result in the development of eating disorders. This is because of the impending temptation to overdo the fast and feast, which eventually negates the benefits that you could have already achieved. This is dangerous in the long run because you can get stuck in the cycle.

Intermittent fasting is not a realistic long-term solution. Just as it is with many other diets, sticking to intermittent fasting, in the long run, can be difficult. A study comparing intermittent fasting to other daily caloric restriction diets established a significant number of dropouts among those who practiced intermittent fasting compared to those who practice calorie cutting. The interesting thing about this study is that most of those who were assigned to the fasting group ended up cutting calories.

Impaired performance in athletes. If you're an athlete, you need to have well-timed fuel to get the most of your work out. Consequently, calorie restriction for extended periods will get in the way of your performance. This will leave you feeling too sluggish even to push the pedal and claim the medal. If you do not time your workout to coincide with your feasting window, then you will also be missing out on muscle growth as well as glycogen replenishment. As a result, you'll end up breaking down your metabolism-boosting muscle instead of building it.

There's little evidence to back it up. Most of the research on intermittent fasting has been done in worms, mice, and rats. Human trials are quite a few; hence, there's not much evidence of the benefits of intermittent fasting in humans. Moreover, studies on the long-term effects of intermittent fasting have not been done. Thus, it is not quite clear if there are any dangers or major benefits that dieters gain in the long run.

You may have cravings. Most of the intermittent fasting protocols will require you to go for long periods without food. The only thing you're free to take is water and unsweetened coffee and tea. Ironically, cravings tend to kick in when you're restricted from eating certain foods. You'll be surprised at how likely you're to crave refined carbs and sweets just because your body is in need of the glucose hit. You'll do well to distract yourself from thinking about food during your fasting window. You can also consider indulging a little during the feeding window so that you satisfy those cravings.

Irritability. It's a common thing to feel a little cranky because of a drop in your blood sugar levels. This can get worse when coupled with other side effects like low energy and cravings. The best way to deal with this is by avoiding people or situations that are likely to make you feel more annoyed and instead focus on the things that will make you happy.

Feeling cold. One of the things you'll experience cold toes and fingers because when you fast, there's an increased flow of blood to your fat stores. This is referred to as the adipose tissue blood flow, which is instrumental in moving fat to your muscles where it's burned as fuel. A decline in the levels of your blood sugar may also be responsible for the increased sensitivity to cold. You can combat this feeling of coldness with hot showers, sipping hot tea, or dressing up in layered clothing. Where possible, stay indoors for longer.

Constipation, heartburn, and bloating. When you eat, your stomach releases acid that is vital in aiding digestion. This means that when you're not eating, you could experience heartburn because there's no food for the acid to act on. Other related complications include burping and mild discomfort. You could also experience pain. These symptoms usually go away on their own over time. All you have to do is make sure you're drinking up sufficient amounts of water and when it's time to eat, avoid the spicy and greasy foods that are likely to worsen the heartburn. Talk to your doctor if it doesn't go away.

Bathroom tips. Since you're taking plenty of water to stay hydrated during fasting, you'll definitely need to make a number of trips to the bathroom. This may be anything from twice an hour. Unfortunately, reducing your water intake may have other side effects; hence, it's better to maintain your water intake.

Overeating. Most people tend to overeat, especially in the initial days of the intermittent fasting journey. This may be because of the misconception that calories don't count in intermittent fasting. The excitement over food leads to overeating. It's important to plan your meals ahead of time so that you stick to eating reasonable portions. Even though you may feel famished at the end of the fasting window, try to eat as normally as you would.

Overreliance on coffee and tea. Most of the intermittent fasting methods you can practice require you to take plenty of water and fluids to stay hydrated and fend off the feeling of hunger. The two most preferred beverages you can take alongside water are tea and coffee. Thus, it's not surprising if you get to a point where you're overly dependent on coffee and tea. Taking too much caffeine can destabilize the quality of your sleep resulting in stress and anxiety that may well promote rebound weight gain.

Feeling too full after eating. When your body gets used to staying without foo over lengthy periods, it affects how you process satiety. You'll begin to realize that eating any snack or a light meal, leaving you feeling too full. This may eventually affect your nutrient intake because then you might end up undereating.

Intermittent fasting presents some not so awesome side effects that you're likely to experience, especially at the beginning. The secret to coping with these side effects is trying to adjust your fasting schedule. In the long run, you must strike a balance

between the benefits and side effects before deciding which way
to go.

Chapter 11: A-Z Glossary

6-Shogoal

The most common of a group of chemicals found in ginger known as shogaols. These chemicals are similar in structure to gingerol. 6-shogaol has been shown to induce autophagy in cancer cells, but not apoptotic cell death.

AMP Kinase

AMP-activated protein kinase is an important enzyme that plays multiple roles in the body, including fatty acid absorption, glucose activation, and oxidation. These processes are part of the larger homeostasis or equilibrium that must be maintained in the body both on a macro level and on a molecular level. AMP-activated protein kinase is sometimes referred to as AMP Kinase or abbreviated as AMPK. AMP Kinase is important in autophagy, and many of the stimulators of autophagy involve activation or increasing concentration of AMP Kinase.

Apoptosis

Pre-programmed cell death. Apoptosis is believed to be regulated by a series of triggers or thresholds that stimulate cells and tissues to initiate the process of cell death. Apoptosis, or programmed cell death, should be distinguished from non-programmed (or non-apoptotic) cell death, of which the most pressing example is autophagy.

ATG

Autophagy-related genes, of which at least 32 are known.

ATP

Adenosine triphosphate, or ATP, is the major energy molecule found in human beings and most other animals. ATP also plays an important role in homeostasis because of the effect that its breakdown and components have in body tissues like the muscles and liver.

Autophagy

A type of non-apoptotic cell death that is regulated by a variety of genes, proteins, and signaling molecules. The name originates from the Greek and it refers to "self-eating." Autophagy is part of the body's normal process of removing components that are superfluous or non-functional, which makes it distinct from the programmed cell death of apoptosis. Autophagy occurs on a cellular and molecular level through the work of proteins, enzymes, and cellular organelles such as the lysosome.

BCAA – Branched Chain Amino Acids

This refers to three amino acids that are essential nutrients which the body obtains from proteins in food. They are; Leucine,

Valine, and Isoleucine. People who have low dietary protein intake can take BCAA supplements to promote muscle protein synthesis and increase the growth of muscle over time.

BMI - Body Mass Index

This is the measure of body fat based on weight and height. It is defined as the body mass that is divided by the square of your body height. The limitation of BMI is that it fails to recognize the muscle or fat of an individual or even their physical build, making it so simplistic.

BMR – Basal Metabolic Rate

This refers to the energy that your body uses when it's at rest. It's aptly defined as the amount of energy expended while at rest in a neutral

Calorie

This is the unit of heat that is used to indicate the amount of energy that different foods will produce in the body. More specifically, a calorie is the amount of heat needed at the pressure of one atmosphere to raise the temperature of a kilogram of water one degree Celsius.

Calorie restriction

This is the practice of consuming fewer calories than the body's Total Daily Energy Expenditure. This leads to weight loss because the body is using more energy than it's receiving.

Cell Death

The general name for the process of destruction of a cell or cellular components. Cell death in the human body is usually divided into apoptotic and non-apoptotic cell death. Autophagy is a type of non-apoptotic cell death, which indicates that though it is carefully regulated it is not programmed in the same manner that apoptosis is.

Chaperone-mediated Autophagy

In this pathway, particles designated for destruction are tagged with a molecule known as a chaperone. The chaperone is there to tag along, alerting the cell's organelles (particularly the lysosome), that this particle is intended for destruction. The particle with the chaperone is recognized by receptors on the lysosomal membrane, which then invaginates the chaperone-tagged particle.

Dry Fasting

The informal name for fasting that is not water fasting.

EGCG

Epigallocatechin gallate, or EGCG, is a catechin found in teas. It is a polyphenol and the most abundant catechin found in tea. Also found in other foods, EGCG has been actively researched because of its potential health benefits. It stimulates autophagy in hepatic cells leading to lipid breakdown. It accomplishes this by increasing the concentration of AMP-activated protein kinase.

Fasting Mimicking Diet

A diet that involves devoting five days out of a 30-day period to a low carbohydrate diet similar to what is seen in the Ketogenic diet. The idea is to "mimic fasting" by shifting the body into Keto during that period so you would basically reap the benefits of a five-day fast even though you actually were eating. During this period, autophagy is used to mobilize fat in hepatic cells and other fat storage areas.

Fasting Window

This is the period through which you will be practicing your fast by abstaining from food.

Feeding Window

This is the time during which you're allowed to eat/ consume calories during intermittent fasting. The duration of the feeding window usually varies depending on the fasting regime.

HGH

Human growth hormone. Human growth hormone is important in bone and organ growth, health and vivacity, and anti-aging. Human growth hormone levels can be increased by fasting, but these effects are only seen in longer periods of fasting.

HIIT

High-intensity interval training. High-intensity interval training has been shown to improve autophagy. High-intensity interval training uses autophagy to stimulate lipolysis (burning of fat).

Intermittent Fasting

A dieting regimen that involves incorporating periods of fasting into your eating schedule. The most common form of intermittent fasting today is a time-limited program in which the day is broken up into periods of fasting and periods of eating. The schedule is divided into hours of fasting and hours of eating. For example, a 16/8 schedule would mean 16 hours of fasting in the day and 8 hours of eating. Most intermittent fasters choose an eating window, such as 12 noon to 8 PM, that works with their commitments and allow them to easily keep track of when they should be fasting and when they are allowed to eat.

Ketogenic Diet

A diet that involves consuming foods that are extremely low in carbohydrates (or have none), which leads to the production of ketone bodies in the liver. The three ketone bodies produced in the liver are acetoacetate, beta-hydroxybutyrate, and acetone. These ketone bodies can be broken down into a molecule called acetyl-CoA and used as a food source. Ketone bodies are known for their characteristic smell, which has been described as fruity.

Ketone Bodies

The name for three bodies produced by the liver when the body has entered "ketosis" as a result of fasting, starvation, disease process, or other conditions. The three ketone bodies produced by the liver are acetoacetate, beta-hydroxybutyrate, and acetone. These are broken down into a molecule called acetyl-CoA and used as energy.

Ketosis

The state of production of ketone bodies in the liver that typically results from long periods of food deprivation as occurs in fasting or starvation. Ketosis involves autophagy, and many diets like the Ketogenic diet have the explicit goal of inducing ketosis. Ketosis is controversial because although this state has some health benefits, it also can result in poor health outcomes if prolonged or associated with a serious condition, such as diabetes mellitus.

LDL

low-density lipoprotein.

Low Carb High Fat

This refers to a dietary system where you consume fewer carbohydrates and instead pack up more fat which you will rely on as your source of energy. Although it sounds counterintuitive since you're actually aiming for far less, it's good for weight loss.

Lysosome

An organelle in the cell that is involved in autophagy through phagocytosis. This organelle works in tandem with other cell organelles, such as the endoplasmic reticulum and the mitochondria to accomplish breakdown of cellular components both as a part of autophagy and outside of it.

Macroautophagy

A process that operates via several steps to trap components in the cytoplasm and recycle them. The first step is the formation of a structure called the isolation membrane. The formation of this structure is triggered by specific factors, some of which will be discussed further shortly. This structure is formed within the cell's cytoplasm; that is, the "sea" of fluid within the cell, as opposed to extracellular fluid outside the cell membrane. Cells are very good at using membranes to separate extracellular components from intracellular ones. This is a means of regulating what is able to enter the cell and protecting the cell.

The second step after the formation of the isolation membrane is the formation of a structure known as the phagophore: a larger structure compared to the initial isolation membrane. The phagophore undergoes a process of expansion which leads to the engulfing of components in the cytoplasm and the formation of a third structure, the autophagosome. The autophagosome may be thought of as the basic essential structure of autophagy. This structure moves towards an important organelle called the lysosome, which results in the fusing of the autophagosome with the lysosome. The result is that the contents of the autophagosome are dumped into the lumen of the lysosome for degradation and recycling.

Macroautophagy is controlled in a highly nuanced manner by a series of triggers. Many of these triggers are in turn signaled and regulated by a number of proteins encoded in genes. Autophagy-related genes, or Atg, refer to proteins involved in the steps that lead to the formation of the autophagosome (via elongation). Triggers of macroautophagy include fasting or starvation, lack of oxygen in the lungs, presence of reactive oxygen species, presence of infectious agents, and therapeutic agents or drugs.

Metabolism
This refers to all the chemical processes that occur in order to maintain the living state of any organism, in this case, the human body.

Microoautophagy
In microoautophagy, the lysosome is the main actor, directly engulfing the components in the cytosol that are intended for degradation. This process involves the double membrane of the lysosome folding in around the components that are being brought into the organelle, a process known as invagination.

Like macroautophagy, this process is stimulated by specific triggers, including various environmental factors

OMAD

One meal a day. Essentially an intermittent fasting diet that involves fasting for 23 hours and eating for one hour a day. Other variations include eating one meal a day every other day, an even longer type of intermittent fasting split.

Phagocytosis

The process of consumption of cell particles, foreign organisms, and debris by lysosomes. Phagocytosis comes from Greek and means "cell eating." It literally refers to the process by which lysosomes, important organelles in the cell, consume and breakdown components with the aid of other organelles, such as the endoplasmic reticulum. This process is generally carefully regulated in the cell with the aid of signaling molecules.

Prebiotic Fiber - foods high in fibers that encourage the growth and maintenance of gut flora. Gut flora is normal bacteria in our GI tract that help us break down food. Examples of prebiotic fiber include artichokes, asparagus, bok choy, and other similar vegetables.

Resistance Training

This is a type of physical exercise involving the use of resistance to induce muscular contraction. It's instrumental in building endurance, strength, and the size of skeletal muscles. Lifting weight is one of the typical forms of resistance training

Telomere Effect - the anti-aging effect that can result from fasting. Increasing telomere length can extend the lifetime of our cells and lead to anti-aging benefits.

Thermic Effect of Food (TEF)

This refers to the amount of energy your body uses when processing and digesting food. It's the main reason for the idea that fasting decreases your metabolism because when you don't eat food, then no energy will be expended in digestion. However, since you haven't eaten any food, it means you haven't taken on any calories altogether. Consequently, eating too many calories to achieve the thermic effect of food to burn off some calories is definitely not a rational decision for weight loss.

Water Fasting

An eating regimen that involves supplanting water for food. So the individual will drink quantities of water as part of their fast.

Frequently Asked Questions About Intermittent Fasting

Here are some of the frequently asked questions about intermittent fasting and their answers:

1. **What is intermittent fasting?**

   Intermittent fasting is a pattern of eating that involves alternating between intervals of fasting and eating. There are different approaches to intermittent fasting as opposed to a one fits all approach.

2. **Will intermittent fasting help me lose weight?**

   One of the benefits of intermittent fasting is fat and weight loss. However, whether you actually get to lose weight is dependent on a number of factors. For instance, if your fasting protocol lets you fast for longer than you have to eat, then you are likely to create a calorie deficit that will drive your weight loss goal. You will also have to watch out that you don't consume processed foods with too many sugars. In short, you will need a shorter fasting window and eat healthy meals to increase weight loss.

3. Can I work out and still practice intermittent fasting?

Of course, yes! It's perfectly safe to practice intermittent fasting and fast. There's evidence to suggest that exercising when fasted may promote fat loss beyond what you'd normally lose when eating normally. Intermittent fasting is designed around when you eat as opposed to restricting calories. Therefore, you can consider aligning your workout schedule to your feeding schedule. Intermittent fasting is an effective way to eat, even for athletes. You'll be surprised to know that that some professional athletes swear by intermittent fasting. If you prefer working out in the morning, you must keep in mind that early morning exercise often sparks big appetite and you don't want to wait for so long before you eat anything.

4. Can I drink tea/coffee while intermittent fasting?

It's okay to have tea/coffee that is unsweetened during intermittent fasting because they have no calories. Sipping on tea or coffee during intermittent fasting is a great way to stay hydrated and focused. Of course, this is in addition to taking water that perhaps the best way to hydrate so that you avoid mindless snacking and feelings of extreme hunger.

5. **How many hours should I fast per day?**

The interesting thing about intermittent fasting is that it doesn't take the 'one fits all approach.' There are different ways through which you can do intermittent fasting. From a minimum of 12 hours of fasting to 48 hours of fasting, you can be sure to find a plan that will meet your needs.

6. **What should I eat when I'm not fasting?**

Fasting offers metabolic health benefits that are independent of what you're eating in your feeding window. Even then, this will not turn the junk food diet into a healthy diet. It's recommended that you eat a healthy balanced diet comprising of carbs, protein, and fats.

7. **Will I lose muscle if I practice intermittent fasting in the long term?**

Like other forms of dietary restriction that result in weight loss, intermittent fasting may cause lean mass and fat loss over time. Even then, there's evidence showing that weight loss that through intermittent fasting may result in less muscle loss and more fat loss compared to caloric restriction and traditional dieting.

8. **Will I feel hungry when fasting?**

It's absolutely normal to feel hungry when fasting. However, you can manage this by drinking plenty of water and other calorie-free drinks to manage your feeling of hunger. Clinical studies have shown that intermittent fasting decreases leptin, the hormone that helps in controlling energy expenditure and increasing experiences of satiety.

9. **Will it be difficult to start intermittent fasting if I'm accustomed to eating or snacking every few hours?**

If you're fasting for the first time, you'll find it to be difficult to transition into this pattern of eating. However, you can be sure to settle into intermittent fasting after a while usually five days. Experts recommend that beginners begin with a larger eating window and gradually lengthen it making the transition much easier.

10.　　　**Should I still fast when I have achieved my ideal body weight?**

Weight loss is not the only benefit of intermittent fasting. This pattern of eating offers other benefits that include increased insulin sensitivity, reduced inflammation, and fat oxidation. This means that you can still fast even when your goal is not to lose weight. However, you'll have to pay attention to how you eat on feast days so that you maintain your weight.

11. Can intermittent fasting help with diabetes?

Research indicates the IF can help in halting the progression of type 2 diabetes. In fact, some doctors suggest that therapeutic fasting can help in eliminating the need for insulin and regulate your blood glucose levels. A report published in the British Medical Journal on men who fasted by consuming few calories on alternate days weaned off insulin injections.

12. Does it matter if I eat early or later in the day?

According to research, the time you eat is as important as the foods you eat. Because of circadian rhythms, insulin sensitivity is at its peak earlier in the day and decreases as the day progresses. When you eat later, it disrupts your circadian rhythm, eventually heightening your risk of type 2 diabetes in the long run. Meals consumed at night usually trigger greater insulin exposure compared to meals that are consumed earlier in the day. Moreover, large bodies of studies have linked nighttime eating to increased risks of cardiovascular disease, cancer, and diabetes.

13.   How do I deal with fatigue or mental fog while fasting?

Intermittent fasting will leave you feeling sluggish and fatigued. The best way to counter this feeling is by drinking up adequate fluids to stay hydrated whether you're fasting or not. Taking coffee will particularly help in boosting your concentration and energy. You can also practice meditation to help you deal with mental fog.

14.   Do I have to stop eating out or attending social gatherings?

One of the benefits of intermittent fasting is flexibility if offers. That is, you get to define when you eat. This helps people to maintain their fasting and eating routines. Even better, you can adjust your eating schedule to fit into your social plans. However, if you occasionally stray, which is a likely situation, you simply get back on track. Although you need to keep enough to keep your health goals in mind, you don't have to be enslaved to them. Remember, intermittent fasting lets you choose a method that works best for you, and this includes your social life.

Is there a best way to break my fast?
The efficacy of post-fast meals on human metabolic health has not been established by scientific studies. However, a number of scientific studies have shown that some people are likely to experience an acute spike in their blood sugar that is linked to insulin resistance after consuming a post-fast meal that is high in carbohydrates. This is more likely to happen in individuals who are not used to extended fasting. If you're new to fasting, you may want to break your fast with meals that are low in glycemic index and high in fiber as well as plant fats. When you get used to fasting, your body will begin experiencing different metabolic reactions to an influx of post-fast nutrients.

15.   Is intermittent fasting safe for me?

Intermittent fasting is beneficial to most people. Even then, there are safety concerns for certain groups of people that include children, pregnant women, and individuals with type 1 diabetes. Individuals who are not getting proper nutrition, as well as those who are malnourished, should also not practice fasting before talking to a doctor. The same goes for young children.

Conclusion

Thank you for making it through the end of *Intermittent Fasting for Women*. Intermittent fasting is a simple yet amazing way to stay healthy and lose weight. Regardless of how much you have tried reaching your weight loss goals in the past, you can be sure to achieve your goals with intermittent fasting.

I believe this has not been another of the many intermittent fasting books, but a real practical guide that will help you get started with your first intermittent fasting experience. But that is just the first step. Intermittent fasting will only provide you great benefits when you practice it in the prescribed manner. You will be surprised at how much of a healthy life you can lead by simply changing your eating pattern.

This book particularly helps you to navigate through intermittent fasting taking, into account the unique nature of the female body that is bound to see a difference in the manner in which your body responds to fasting. It also captures why most women always find it difficult losing weight despite trying out all kinds of diets. This book is an excellent resource since it covers all the information you need to know. From the benefits of intermittent fasting to what you need to do to transition smoothly and even the myths and common mistakes you can make with this program.

Therefore, you'll do well to go back in the book and make reference any area whenever you need a clarification. This will catapult you to success with this pattern of eating.